The 5-Minute
Child
Health
Advisor

Derived from The 5 Minute Pediatric Consult

M. WILLIAM SCHWARTZ, MD
EDITOR

ASSOCIATE DIRECTORS
LOUIS M. BELL, MD
PETER M. BINGHAM, MD
ESTHER K. CHUNG, MD
DAVID R. FRIEDMAN, MD
ANDREW E. MULBERG, MD
LAURA N. SINAI, MD

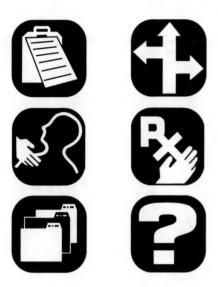

The 5-Minute Child Health Advisor

EDITOR
M. WILLIAM SCHWARTZ, MD
PROFESSOR OF PEDIATRICS
ASSOCIATE DEAN OF PRIMARY CARE EDUCATION
UNIVERSITY OF PENNSYLVANIA SCHOOL OF MEDICINE
CHILDREN'S HOSPITAL OF PHILADELPHIA
PHILADELPHIA, PENNSYLVANIA

Consulting Author
BRUCE GOLDFARB

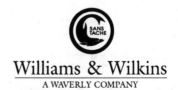

Williams & Wilkins
A WAVERLY COMPANY

BALTIMORE • PHILADELPHIA • LONDON • PARIS • BANGKOK
BUENOS AIRES • HONG KONG • MUNICH • SYDNEY • TOKYO • WROCLAW

Editor: David Charles Retford
Managing Editor: Jennifer Eckhoff
Marketing Manager: Daniell T. Griffin
Production Coordinator: Marette D. Magargle-Smith
Project Editor: Kathy Gilbert
Cover Designer: Graphic World, Inc.
Typesetter: Peirce Graphic Services, Inc.
Printer & Binder: Victor Graphics, Inc.

Printed in the United States of America

First Edition,

Library of Congress Cataloging-in-Publication Data

The 5 minute child health advisor / editor, M. William Schwartz ;
  consulting editor, Bruce Goldfarb.
    p. cm.
  Includes index.
  ISBN 0–683–30433–X
  1. Pediatrics—Popular works. 2. Children—Health and hygiene.
3. Children—Disease. I. Schwartz, M. Williams, 1935– .
II. Goldfarb, Bruce.
RJ61.A13   1997
618.92—dc21   97-24983
                                   CIP

To purchase additional copies of this book, please call our customer service department at **(800) 638-0672** or fax orders to **(800) 447-8438.** For other book services, including chapter reprints and large quantity sales, ask for the Special Sales department.

Canadian customers should call **(800) 665-1148,** or fax **(800) 665-0103.** For all other calls originating outside of the United States, please call **(401) 528-4223** or fax us at **(410) 528-8550.**

Visit Williams & Wilkins on the Internet: **http://www.wwilkins.com** or contact our customer service department at **custserv@wwilkins.com.** Williams & Wilkins customer service representatives are available from 8:30 am to 6:00 pm, EST, Monday through Friday, for telephone access.

97 98 99 00
2 3 4 5 6 7 8 9 10

Dedication

This book for parents is dedicated to my parents, Harry Schwartz, that rare combination of a scholarly Southern Gentleman and Yankee Trader, and Sylvia Schwartz, whose energy taught me how to do ten things at once. Both instilled in their children a love of books, respect for tradition and a life of integrity.

It is also dedicated to my in-laws Robert Goldner, who personified the gentle gentleman and Pearl C. Goldner, a wonderful example of modern elegance, whose energy and vision has made life better for many people.

Preface

When the proposal to develop *The 5 Minute Child Health Advisor* arose, the first thought I had was: "what a great idea for parents!" Now the book is a reality. In this age of information and informed patients, this publication contributes to better patient care by explaining to parents what their child has or does not have. Too often, lack of information leads to unnecessary worry and unproductive behavior. Efforts such as this book attempt to enlighten parents so that they can learn about children's health issues as well as enjoy their children more by worrying less. I have been impressed by how often the presence of a common problem such as bruises makes leukemia, not trauma, highest on the parents' worry list. By having information about bruises, trauma and leukemia, we hope some anxieties may be relieved.

What this book is and what it is not. *The 5 Minute Child Health Advisor* has been called "a book of the nineties," meaning that the format presents information quickly and concisely. In today's parlance, it is a database, meaning important information on some 200 diseases can be accessed quickly. Other components include a list of syndromes and tables of normal and abnormal data. Information . . . Information . . . Information. . . .

What it is not, is a license to diagnosis and treat. It is not a guide to evaluate and manage your child independently; these tasks take more than data and questions. They require experience, interpretive skills, weighing of conflicting data, judgment and decision making. Such activities are not addressed in this book.

Books like this take a great deal of teamwork. In this case it started with an idea from the editorial leadership which turned into a call "what do you think about this idea?" Then, with the audience in mind, topics were selected for inclusion into the final product. Next the team is organized, with the overlying principle that the job should be fun. Many people were eager to contribute for various reasons, as publications such as this help them put their ideas into an organized format to teach others; on another level, the authors need to publish articles and chapters as part of the promotion process. Therein lies the editor's dilemma: Many eager writers do well. Many write too much and too late. Selection of the former over the latter is part luck and part experience. These talented writers make the book what it is. They have done an excellent job.

My thanks to the staff of Williams & Wilkins for their expertise and cooperation. Special appreciation to Jennifer Eckhoff for her organizational skills and efforts to produce this book. For this edition, Bruce Goldfarb rewrote the text, taking what was written for a medical audience and redirecting to you the parents. We hope you like it and use it wisely.

Contributors

Unless otherwise indicated, faculty appointments are at the University of Pennsylvania School of Medicine, and hospital appointments are at Children's Hospital of Philadelphia, Pennsylvania.

Sotiria C. Apostolopoulou, M.D.
Cardiologist
Athens, Greece

Linda D. Arnold, M.D.
Division of Gastroenterology

Mark L. Bagarazzi, M.D.
Fellow, Infectious Disease
Instructor in Pediatrics

Meena Scavena Baldi, D.O.
Neurologist
Alfred I. Dupont Institute
Wilmington, Delaware

Louis M. Bell, M.D.
Associate Professor of Pediatrics
Attending Physician
Departments of Infectious Diseases and
    Emergency Medicine

A.G. Christina Bergqvist, M.D.
Fellow, Child Neurology
Instructor in Pediatrics

Lisa M. Biggs, M.D.
Instructor
Primary Care Center

Peter M. Bingham, M.D.
Assistant Professor of Neurology in
    Pediatrics
Assistant Physician, Department of
    Pediatrics

Nathan J. Blum, M.D.
Assistant Professor of Pediatrics
Division of Child Development and
    Rehabilitation
The Children's Seashore House.

Amy R. Brooks-Kayal, M.D.
Assistant Professor
Departments of Neurology and Pediatrics
Attending Neurologist

James M. Callahan, M.D.
Assistant Professor of Pediatrics
Department of Pediatrics and Emergency
    Medicine
Syracuse University Medical Center

William B. Carey, M.D.
Director, Section on Behavioral Pediatrics
Division of General Pediatrics
Clinical Professor of Pediatrics

Christine A. Carman-Dillon, M.D.
Resident, Plastic Surgery

Rosemary Casey, M.D.
Assistant Professor of Pediatrics
Thomas Jefferson University
Main Line Pediatrics

Suzette Surratt Caudle, M.D.
Attending Physician
Division of General Pediatrics
Department of Pediatrics
Carolinas Medical Center
Charlotte, North Carolina

Elizabeth Candell Chalom, M.D.
Fellow, Pediatric Rheumatology

Cindy W. Christian, M.D.
Assistant Professor of Pediatrics
Medical Director, Child Abuse Services

Esther K. Chung, M.D., M.P.H.
Instructor in Pediatrics
Fellow, General Pediatrics

Liana R. Clark, M.D.
Clinical Assistant Professor
Department of General Pediatrics
Section of Adolescent Medicine

Contributors

Susan E. Coffin, M.D.
Instructor
Division of Allergy, Immunology and
    Infectious Diseases

Mitchell I. Cohen, M.D.
Fellow
Pediatric Cardiology

Paulo Collett-Solberg, M.D.
Fellow
Division of Endocrinology

Richard S. Davidson, M.D.
Associate Professor of Orthopaedic Surgery
Attending Surgeon, Division of
    Orthopaedic Surgery

Susan Dibs, M.D.
Assistant Professor of Pediatrics
Yale New Haven Medical Center

Dennis J. Dlugos, M.D.
Fellow, Child Neurology
Instructor in Pediatrics

Joel A. Fein, M.D.
Assistant Professor of Pediatrics
University of Pennsylvania School of
    Medicine
Attending Physician
Emergency Department

Hector L. Flores-Arroyo, M.D.
Division of Pulmonary Medicine

Jill A. Foster, M.D.
Assistant Professor of Pediatrics
Allegheny University of the Health Sciences
Attending Physician
St. Christopher's Hospital for Children
Philadelphia, Pennsylvania

Janet H. Friday, M.D.
Emergency Department
Connecticut Children's Hospital

Debra L. Friedman, M.D.
Fellow
Division of Hematology-Oncology

James B. Gibson, M.D.
Assistant Professor of Pediatrics
Section of Genetics
University of Arkansas for Medical Science
Little Rock, Arkansas

Kenneth R. Ginsburg, M.D.
Assistant Professor of Pediatrics
Section of Adolescent Medicine
Department of Pediatrics

Pilar Gonzalez-Serrano, M.D.
Fellow, Pulmonary Medicine
Instructor in Pediatrics

Marc H. Gorelick, M.D.
Assistant Professor of Pediatrics and
    Epidemiology
Attending Physician
Division of Pediatric Emergency
    Medicine

Cynthia Guzzo, M.D.
Associate Professor
Department of Dermatology

Barbara Haber, M.D.
Assistant Professor of Pediatrics
Division of Gastroenterology and Nutrition

Hakon Hakonarson, M.D.
Assistant Professor of Pediatrics
Assistant Physician, Pulmonary Medicine

Virginia Moodey Hamilton, M.D.
Hematology Fellow
Department of Pediatrics

Cheryl Hausman, M.D.
Director of General Pediatrics
Albert Einstein Medical Center
Philadelphia, Pennsylvania

Michael D. Hogarty, M.D.
Divisions of Hematology and Oncology

Douglas Hyder, M.D.
Department of Neurology
Children's Hospital of Los Angeles
Los Angeles, California

Helen John, M.D.
Division of Gastroenterology and Nutrition

Robert Kamei, M.D.
Associate Professor of Clinical Pediatrics
Division of General Pediatrics
Department of Pediatrics
University of California-San Francisco
San Francisco, California

Aaron S. Kaplan, D.O.
Assistant Professor of Pediatrics
Section of Pediatric Gastroenterology and
    Nutrition
Tulane Medical School
New Orleans, Louisiana

Lorraine Katz, M.D.
Assistant Professor
Division of Endocrinology and Diabetes

Gregory F. Keenan, M.D.
Assistant Professor of Pediatrics
Section of Rheumatology

Kara M. Kelly, M.D.
Assistant Professor of Pediatrics
College of Physicians and Surgeons of
    Columbia University
Attending Physician, Pediatric Oncology
Columbia-Presbyterian Medical Center
New York, New York

Michelle M. Klinek, M.D.
Allergy and Asthma Consultants
York, Pennsylvania

Deborah L. Kramer, M.D.
Fellow, Child Hematology/Oncology
Instructor in Pediatrics

Richard Mark Kravitz, M.D.
Assistant Professor of Pediatrics
Division of Pulmonary Medicine
Department of Pediatrics

Jane Lavelle, M.D.
Assistant Professor of Pediatrics
Division of Pediatric Emergency Medicine
Associate Physician, Emergency Medicine

Mary B. Leonard, M.D.
Associate Professor of Pediatrics

Grant T. Liu, M.D.
Assistant Professor
Departments of Neurology and
    Ophthalmology
Scheie Eye Institute

David W. Low, M.D.
Assistant Professor of Surgery
Division of Plastic Surgery

Jacalyn S. Maller, M.D.
Clinical Assistant Professor of Pediatrics
Assistant Physician
Divisions of Emergency Medicine and
    General Pediatrics

Eric S. Maller, M.D.
Assistant Professor of Pediatrics
Medical Director, Liver Transplant Program
Division of Gastroenterology and
    Nutrition

Maria R. Mascarenhas, M.D.
Assistant Professor of Pediatrics
Division of Gastroenterology and Nutrition
Department of Pediatrics
Director, Nutrition Support Services

Christina Master, M.D.
Chief Resident Physician
Instructor in Pediatrics

D. Elizabeth McNeil, M.D.
Fellow, Child Neuro-oncology
Instructor in Pediatrics

Kevin E.C. Meyers, M.D.
Division of Nephrology

Patricia T. Molloy, M.D.
Assistant Professor of Neurology
Instructor in Pediatrics

Thomas Moshang, Jr., M.D.
Professor of Pediatrics
Senior Physician
Director of Endocrinology

Contributors

Christen Mowad, M.D.
Assistant Professor of Dermatology
Department of Dermatology

Andrew E. Mulberg, M.D.
Assistant Professor of Pediatrics

Roberto Nachajon, M.D.
Fellow, Pulmonary Medicine
Instructor in Pediatrics

Michael N. Needle, M.D.
Assistant Professor
Division of Oncology
Department of Pediatrics

Kevin C. Osterhoudt, M.D.
Fellow, Emergency Medicine/Toxicology
Instructor in Pediatrics

Yvonne Paris, M.D.
Fellow
Division of Cardiology

Carmen M. Parrott, M.D.
Fellow
Department of Dermatology

Louis Pelligrino, M.D.
Assistant Professor
Assistant Physician
Children's Seashore House

David A. Piccoli, M.D.
Associate Professor of Pediatrics
Interim Chief
Division of Gastroenterology
   and Nutrition

Bret Rudy, M.D.
Assistant Professor of Pediatrics
Assistant Physician, General Pediatrics

Richard M. Rutstein, M.D.
Assistant Professor of Pediatrics
Medical Director, Special Immunology
   Service
Division of General Pediatrics

Marta Satin-Smith, M.D.
Assistant Professor of Pedicatics
Eastern VA School of Medicine

David B. Schaffer, M.D.
Professor of Ophthalmology
Chairman, Division of Ophthalmology

Seth L. Schulman, M.D.
Assistant Professor of Pediatrics
Division of Pediatric Nephrology

Philip V. Scribano, D.O.
Assistant Professor of Pediatric
   Emergency Medicine
University of Connecticut
Farmington, Connecticut

Edisio Semeao, M.D.
Fellow, Division of Gastroenterology

Sadhna M. Shankar, M.D.
Fellow, Cardiology
Instructor in Pediatrics

Kathy N. Shaw, M.D.
Associate Professor of Pediatrics
Acting Division Chief, Emergency
   Department

Deborah L. Silver, M.D.
Clinical Assistant Professor
Associate Director
Children's Hospital/Abington Memorial
   Pediatric Service
Abington, Pennsylvania

Laura N. Sinai, M.D.
Clinical Affiliate
Division of General Pediatrics

Christopher A. Smith, M.D.
Fellow, Allergy and Immunology
Instructor in Pediatrics

Kim Smith-Whitley, M.D.
Assistant Professor of Pediatrics
Assistant Physician
Division of Hematology

Molly W. Stevens, M.D.
Assoc. Professor of Pediatrics
Division of Emergency Medicine

Catherine B. Sullivan, M.D.
Clinical Staff Associate
Department of Pediatrics

Olafur Thorarenson, M.D.
Fellow, Neurology
Instructor in Pediatrics

Nicholas Tsarouhas, M.D.
Assistant Professor of Clinical Pediatrics
    and Surgery
Robert Wood Johnson Medical School
Director, Pediatric Emergency Medicine
Camden, New Jersey

Takeshi Tsuda, M.D.
Fellow, Cardiology
Instructor in Pediatrics

John Tung, M.B.B.S., M.R.C.P. (UK)
Fellow
Division of Pediatric Gastroenterology

Sheila N. Vaughan, R.N., B.S.N.
Division of Neurology

Emily von Scheven, M.D.
Assistant Clinical Professor of Pediatrics
Section of Pediatric Rheumatology
Department of Pediatrics
University of California-San Francisco
San Francisco, California

Dror Wasserman, M.D.
Fellow, Gastroenterology
Instructor in Pediatrics

Barbara Watson, M.D.
Medical Immunization Specialist
Division of Disease Control
Philadelphia Department of Public Health
Philadelphia, Pennsylvania

Stuart A. Weinzimer, M.D.
Fellow, Endocrinology
Instructor in Pediatrics

William J. Wenner, Jr., M.D.
Assistant Professor of Pediatrics
Division of Gastroenterology
    and Nutrition
Attending Gastroenterologist

Therese B. West, M.D.
Clinical Associate in Pediatrics

Catherine C. Wiley, M.D.
Clinical Assistant Professor
    of Pediatrics
Department of Pediatrics
University of Connecticut School of
    Medicine
Farmington, Connecticut
Attending Pediatrician
Connecticut Children's Medical Center
Hartford, Connecticut

Martin C. Wilson, M.D.
Department of Ophthalmology

George Anthony Woodward, M.D.
Assistant Professor of Pediatrics
Division of Emergency Medicine
Medical Director, Section of Transport
    Medicine
Attending Physician,
    Emergency Department

Donna Zeiter, M.D.
Hartford Children's Hospital
Hartford, Connecticut

Kathy Wholey Zsolway, D.O.
Assistant Professor of Pediatrics

Contents

Section I: What You Need to Know About . . . / 1

Contents

SECTION II: Definitions / 327

Contents

The 5-Minute Child Health Advisor

SECTION I:
What You Need to Know About...

Acre

 Basics

DESCRIPTION

Acne is a common disorder of the sebaceous glands that predominantly affects adolescents. Pimple lesions may become inflamed and reddened.

SIGNS AND SYMPTOMS

- Pimples, blackheads, whiteheads, nodules, and cysts
- Usually affects the face, but the chest, back, thighs, buttocks, and upper arms can also be affected. Acne spares the hands, forearms, calves, feet, and armpits.

CAUSES

- Blockage of sebaceous ducts in skin
- Hormones
- Bacteria
- Fats
- Abnormal skin growth
- Stress/fatigue

SCOPE

Acne is common among adolescents.

 Diagnosis

QUESTIONS THE DOCTOR WILL ASK

- Diet?
- Rest?
- Stress?
- Soaps?
- Treatment?
- Sun exposure?
- Washing of face procedures?
- Relation to menstrual cycle?

WHAT THE DOCTOR LOOKS FOR

- The doctor will determine the types of lesions present, number of each type, intensity of in-flammation, extent of pigmentation changes of the skin, and scarring.
- Distribution of lesions on body
- Pressure of cysts

TESTS AND PROCEDURES

- Skin may be cultured.
- Adolescent girls with severe acne may be checked for hormone disorders.

 Treatment

GENERAL MEASURES

- Acne is not caused by dirt or oil on the surface of the skin. The skin should be washed gently with a mild soap. Frequent, vigorous washing or excessive scrubbing of the face with abrasives is unnecessary and may lead to a dermatitis.
- Astringents and rubbing alcohol make the skin's surface less oily but have minimal bene-ficial effect on the acne. They may irritate the skin.

ACTIVITY

N/A

DIET

Cola, chocolate, sweets, milk, ice cream, shellfish, nuts, and fatty foods have not been shown to have any effect on severity of acne.

 Medications

COMMONLY PRESCRIBED DRUGS

- Benzoyl peroxide
- Tretinoin (Retin A)
- Other exfoliates: Washes and lotions usually contain salicylic acid, resorcinol, sulfur, or phenol; abrasive scrubs contain almond shells, aluminum oxide, or pumice.
- Erythromycin, clindamycin (topical)
- Antibiotics (oral)
- Isotretinoin (Accutane)

Follow-Up

WHAT TO EXPECT

- Superficial lesions will heal in 5 to 10 days with little scarring.
- Deep papules usually have more intense inflammation and can take weeks to resolve. There may also be scarring.
- Antibiotics should be tapered and discontinued as soon as possible after healing.
- Improvement is seen after 4 to 6 weeks of therapy.
- Acne improves with age, but 5–10% of young adults still report significant acne.

SIGNS TO WATCH

- Worsening of acne lesions
- Scarring and changes in skin pigmentation

PREVENTION

- Lesions must not be picked at or squeezed: this may result in scarring.
- Stress may make acne worse; stress relaxation techniques should be used for adolescents with high stress levels.

 ## Common Questions and Answers

Q: What types of soaps should those with acne use?
A: Acne-prone skin does not need the many harsh scrubs and cleansers that are found on the market. Antibacterial soaps are not necessary. It is best to use a gentle cleansing soap such as Dove, Neutrogena, or Purpose twice a day. Washing with the fingertips is best, rather than using a scrubbing pad or washcloth.

Q: What advice should be given those undergoing acne treatment?
A: It is important that the adolescent be patient during therapy. It often takes 4–6 weeks before one sees visible results. They should also avoid picking at or squeezing any pimples. This may result in scarring. Also make sure that they use makeup and moisturizers that don't cause acne.

Q: Does the acne have to be moderate to severe to use tretinoin (Retin A)?
A: Actually, tretinoin is one of the best topical medications to use for mild acne. It should be used every other night for a week and if there is no irritation, it can be increased to every night. It is important that tretinoin not be used in the daytime. Retin A causes peeling of skin and redness. Also, sunscreens with an SPF greater than 15 should be used if the time is spent outdoors.

Adenovirus Infection

 Basics

DESCRIPTION

Adenoviruses are common viruses that most often cause upper respiratory symptoms. These viruses may also affect the throat, eyes, gastrointestinal tract, or other body systems.

SIGNS AND SYMPTOMS

- Fever
- Reddened eyes
- Rhinitis
- Laryngitis, sore throat
- Rapid breathing rate, wheezing
- Nonproductive or croupy cough
- Headache, muscle ache
- Hematuria (gross or microscopic), dysuria, urinary frequency
- Abdominal tenderness, distension
- Watery diarrhea

CAUSES

Viral infection

SCOPE

- Infection usually occurs early in life (usually by 10 years of age) and is most often characterized by upper respiratory symptoms.
- Respiratory and intestinal infections may occur at any time of year. Epidemics of respiratory disease occur in winter and spring.
- Outbreaks of infection have been associated with inadequately chlorinated swimming pools.
- Military recruits are especially susceptible to infection, probably because of crowded living conditions.

 Diagnosis

QUESTIONS THE DOCTOR MAY ASK

When it started, any contact with sick people, treatment, symptoms

WHAT THE DOCTOR LOOKS FOR

Signs and symptoms of the throat, respiratory system, and gastrointestinal tract.

TESTS AND PROCEDURES

- Usually none required
- Blood tests
- Chest x-ray
- Viral culture, isolation, and identification

Treatment

GENERAL MEASURES

Prevent spread of infection by washing hands frequently.

ACTIVITY

No limitation

DIET

Regular. Encourage fluids

 ## Medications

COMMONLY PRESCRIBED DRUGS

Treat fever with fluids and acetaminophen or ibuprofen.

 ## Follow-Up

WHAT TO EXPECT

Outcome is usually good; most cases are self-limiting.

SIGNS TO WATCH:

• Persistence of illness

PREVENTION

• Body fluids caution
• Oral vaccines have been used by the military.

 ## Common Questions and Answers

Q: How did I get it?
A: Contact with another person.

Q: How can it be avoided?
A: You can't always avoid it. Shower, wash hands, and avoid crowds during high incidence times.

Anaerobic Infection

Basics

DESCRIPTION

Anaerobes are organisms capable of growing in a low-oxygen environment. They pose an increased risk to those with an impaired immune system or devitalized tissue (caused by surgery, trauma, or vascular insufficiency).

SIGNS AND SYMPTOMS

- Formation of pus
- Abscess formation
- Tissue destruction

CAUSES

Bacteria such as clostridia, bacteroides, and gram-negative aneroibes.

SCOPE

- Less frequent in children than in adults
- Responsible for up to 10% of significant bacteria-related episodes in infants and children

Diagnosis

QUESTIONS THE DOCTOR MAY ASK

- Trauma
- Recent surgery
- Exposure to sick people

WHAT THE DOCTOR LOOKS FOR

- Location of infection
- Poor dentition
- Putrid odor
- Gas in tissue
- Pus

TESTS AND PROCEDURES

- Culture and identification of bacteria
- X-rays
- Special imaging studies: computed tomography (CT) and/or magnetic resonance imaging (MRI)

Treatment

GENERAL MEASURES

- Drug therapy
- Surgery may be required for drainage of abscesses and debridement of devitalized tissue.
- Hyperbaric (pressurized) oxygen

ACTIVITY

Limitation depends on location of infection.

DIET

N/A

 ## Medications

COMMONLY PRESCRIBED DRUGS

Antibiotics: cefotaxime, metronidazole, oxacillin, chloramphenicol, penicillin, clindamycin, ampicillin, sulbactam, cefoxitin, gentamicin

 ## Follow-Up

WHAT TO EXPECT

- The outcome is determined by the speed with which infection is appropriately treated.
- Up to 40% death rate is associated with severe anaerobic bacterial infection.

SIGNS TO WATCH

Increasing size of infected area

PREVENTION

N/A

 ## Common Questions and Answers

N/A

Anaphylaxis

Basics

DEFINITION

Anaphylaxis is an explosive allergic reaction.

SIGNS AND SYMPTOMS

- Rash and swelling of skin
- Spasm, swelling of the airway, wheezing
- Swelling may be noted anywhere but is more significant if it involves the lips, tongue, mouth, or throat.
- Profusely runny nose
- Nausea, vomiting, diarrhea, gastrointestinal pain
- Rapid or irregular heart rhythm
- Shock

CAUSES

- Antibiotics (penicillin and others)
- Foreign proteins (bee sting venom, latex, fire ant venom, and others)
- Therapeutic agents (allergen extracts, measles-mumps-rubella [MMR] vaccine, drugs, and others)
- Foods (peanuts, nuts, shellfish, and others)

SCOPE

- Annual incidence of 0.4 case per million individuals.
- 400 to 800 deaths annually in the United States
- Allergies can run in families.

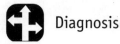

Diagnosis

QUESTIONS THE DOCTOR MAY ASK

- Have you ever had anaphylaxis in the past?
- Did you self-administer epinephrine?
- Have you been stung by a bee, or are you allergic to any foods?
- Do you have asthma or heart disease?

WHAT THE DOCTOR LOOKS FOR

- Reactions usually begin within seconds to minutes after contact with offending substance, but may take longer to evolve.
- Patient must have had previous exposure to the offending allergen for sensitization to occur.
- Patient may have an initial sense of impending doom.
- Target organs are rapidly affected (cardiovascular, respiratory, skin, and gastrointestinal).
- Death may result from asphyxiation from upper airway obstruction or profound shock or both.

TESTS AND PROCEDURES

- The treatment of anaphylaxis should never be withheld while awaiting laboratory confirmation.
- Blood tests
- Chest X-ray
- Electrocardiogram (EKG)

Treatment

GENERAL MEASURES

- Provide emergency first aid as needed, including rescue breathing.
- Health care personnel may apply a tourniquet to decrease the amount of toxin-containing blood circulating from the site of stings and injections.
- Oxygenate, place in recumbent position, and elevate legs.
- Intravenous (IV) fluids and drugs
- Patients not admitted to the hospital should be observed for several hours because some reactions can begin as late as 12 hours after the initial anaphylaxis. These patients are at risk for a second episode of anaphylaxis.
- All patients who have had anaphylaxis should be given epinephrine in an auto-injecting apparatus.
- Patients with a known trigger should be counseled on strict avoidance.
- All patients should have a follow-up visit with an allergist.

ACTIVITY

Use auto-injector if spending time out of doors.

DIET

Avoid foods and substances known to trigger allergies.

 ## Medications

COMMONLY PRESCRIBED DRUGS

Epinephrine

 ## Follow-Up

WHAT TO EXPECT

The outcome is excellent as long as the trigger can be avoided.

SIGNS TO WATCH

Seek immediate medical help if symptoms return.

PREVENTION

Avoid substances that cause allergies.

 ## Common Questions and Answers

Q: When should the auto-injectable epinephrine be used?
A: It is intended for severe allergic reactions as manifested by any of the following: bronchospasm, swelling of the lips or tongue, or hypotension (dizziness). The patient must seek immediate medical help if the auto-injectable epinephrine is required.

Q: Do patients outgrow this condition?
A: No. Subsequent reactions tend to have a more rapid onset, and tend to be more severe.

Q: Who should be referred to an allergist?
A: All patients who have experienced anaphylaxis would benefit from consultation with an allergist. Patients with anaphylaxis from bee stings and certain antibiotics can be desensitized. Furthermore, the allergist can be helpful in identifying obscure triggers of anaphylaxis.

Anemia, Hemolytic

 Basics

DEFINITION

Anemia is characterized by shortened red blood cell survival.

SIGNS AND SYMPTOMS

- Pallor
- Jaundice
- Dark urine
- Fever
- Weakness
- Dizziness
- Fainting
- Dizziness upon standing

CAUSES

- Idiopathic (unknown)
- Infection—malaria
- Drug reaction—sulfa
- Food (Fava beans)
- Transfer of maternal antibodies
- Destruction of cells by spleen (sickle cell anemia)
- Defect of red cells (GGPD)

SCOPE

- Less common in children and adolescents than in adults
- Peak incidence in childhood is in first 4 years of life.
- Death rate in children ranges from 9 to 19%.

 Diagnosis

WHAT THE DOCTOR LOOKS FOR

- Paleness
- Jaundice
- Enlargement of liver or spleen
- Acute disease
- Weakness
- Renal failure
- Onset with rapid fall in hemoglobin level over hours to days
- Usual course: complete resolution of disease within 3 to 6 months
  - Resolution more likely in children who present between 2 and 12 years of age
- Chronic disease
  - Slower onset of anemia over weeks to months, with some having persistent hemolysis or intermittent relapses
  - More likely to be associated with underlying disorder
  - More common in adults and children younger than 2 years or older than 12 years

TESTS AND PROCEDURES

- Blood tests (CBC, coombs test)
- Urinalysis
- Bone marrow may be sampled.

Treatment

GENERAL MEASURES

- Blood transfusion (if needed)
- Oral medication

ACTIVITY

Reset until the hemoglobin level is stabilized.

DIET

N/A

Medications

COMMONLY PRESCRIBED DRUGS

- Usually none required
- Corticosteroids: prednisone, methylpred-nisolone
- Intravenous immune globulin (IVIG)
- Immune suppressive agents

 ## Follow-Up

WHAT TO EXPECT

Outcome depends on age, underlying disorder (if any), and response to therapy.

SIGNS TO WATCH

- Progress to chronic anemia
- Enlargement of spleen

PREVENTION

Avoid food (fava beans) or drugs (antibiotics) that may cause anemia

 ## Common Questions and Answers

Q: How long does acute hemolytic anemia last?
A: 3–6 months in typical course.

Q: When is removal of spleen indicated in chronic hemolytic anemia?
A: If patient is unresponsive to medical management; those requiring high dosage of steroids.

Angioedema

Basics

DESCRIPTION

Angioedema is an inherited disorder that results in a tendency to develop severe swelling. Angioedema may occur in the upper airway, gastrointestinal tract, and extremities. Life-threatening upper airway obstruction may develop.

CAUSES

- Inherited genetic defect
- Allergic reactions (food, inhalation, ingestion, contact)
- Drug reaction
- Panic attacks
- Rash (e.g., cold rash, sun rash, water rash)
- Exercise-induced anaphylaxis
- Pressure or vibration
- Hereditary vibratory angioedema
- Transfusion reaction
- Vascular disease
- Angiotensin-converting enzyme (ACE) inhibitors
- Unknown

SCOPE

N/A

Diagnosis

QUESTIONS THE DOCTOR MAY ASK

- Do you have a family history of similar symptoms?
- Do hives develop with these attacks?
- What are your triggers for attacks?
- When did your attacks begin, and are they getting more frequent?
- Do your attacks respond to epinephrine, antihistamines, and corticosteroids?
- Do you have other medical problems (cancer)?

WHAT THE DOCTOR LOOKS FOR

- Life-threatening upper airway obstruction
- Recurrent attacks of subcutaneous swelling that usually begin around puberty
- Attacks are characterized by swelling of the upper airway, extremities, or bowels (causes severe abdominal pain).
- Attacks are *not* associated with hives.
- Attacks last 1–4 days.
- Attacks are triggered by emotional stress and physical trauma.
- Usually family history of similar symptoms
- Attacks respond poorly to epinephrine, antihistamines, and corticosteroids.
- Severe abdominal pain often mistaken for a surgical abdomen (e.g., appendicitis)
- Aside from angioedema, the physical examination is normal.

TESTS AND PROCEDURES

Blood tests

Treatment

GENERAL MEASURES

- Treatment of the underlying cause often results in resolution of the angioedema.
- Preventive medication (steroids)
- Management of acute episodes

DIET

N/A

ACTIVITY

N/A

Medications

COMMONLY PRESCRIBED DRUGS

- Anabolic steroids (danazol or stanozolol)
- Plasmin inhibitors (e-aminocaproic acid or tranexamic acid)
- Epinephrine
- C1-INH concentrate

 ## Follow-Up

WHAT TO EXPECT

- Patients should be seen at least annually.
- Follow-up should be with an endocrinologist when patients are placed on androgen therapy.
- Follow-up should include a review of triggers, prospective genetic counseling when appropriate, reinforcement of the need for prevention, and review of attacks during the previous year.
- Attacks may be triggered by minor trauma, especially dental procedures.
- Outcome is good with preventive therapy.

SIGNS TO WATCH

N/A

PREVENTION

N/A

 ## Common Questions and Answers

Q: When should a child with angioedema be referred to an immunologist?
A: Recurrent angioedema that begins around puberty should raise the suspicion of hereditary angioedema. If the family has a history of angioedema, if the angioedema is associated with abdominal pain, or if the angioedema is triggered by trauma, the patient should be referred to an immunologist. Hereditary angioedema is not associated with hives or rash. If the patient also has hives with the angioedema, the cause is not hereditary angioedema.

Q: What are the side effects of the prophylactic medication (drugs to prevent episodes)?
A: The prophylactic medication is anabolic steroids. Side effects include masculinization, menstrual irregularities, stunted bone growth, water retention, hypertension, hepatitis, liver cancer, decreased sperm production, and gynecomastia.

Q: Over what period of time may acute angioedema recur?
A: Six weeks, with each episode lasting approximately a period of hours.

Q: What kinds of things may lead to an episode of angioedema?
A: Food allergy, food additives, drugs (antibiotics, aspirin, vaccines), insect stings, physical exposure (heat, cold, exercise) thyroid disease, diabetes mellitus, systemic lupus erythematosus (SLE), multiple infections, contact allergy (animals, latex).

Animal Bites and Stings

 Basics

DESCRIPTION

Dogs are responsible for 90 to 95% of cases of animal bites, while the remainder of cases are divided as follows: cats, 3–8%; rodents or rabbits, 1%; and raccoons and other animals, 1%. Ninety percent of the offending animals are well-known to the victim.

- Although fatalities from animal bites are rare, the majority of them occur in the pediatric population.
- Ten percent of animal bites require suturing, 5–50% develop into infections, 30% cause disability, and 50% leave scars.
- Although there are approximately 20,000 species of venomous spiders in the United States, most lack fangs capable of penetrating human skin or toxin strong enough to produce more than a mild reaction.
- Two species of spiders, however, can cause significant harm. The black, red, and brown widow spiders (Latrodectus species) and brown recluse spiders (Loxosceles species) can cause severe local and systemic reactions, including death.
- Although there are approximately 120 snake species in this country, only 15% produce poisonous substances capable of causing fatal reactions.
- Approximately 8000 people annually in the United States sustain a poisonous snakebite, and 12–15 fatalities occur.
- Four of 20 species of poisonous snakes found in North America are responsible for the majority of bites: Crotalidae (pit viper family: rattlesnakes, cottonmouths, copperheads), and Elapidae (coral snakes).

SIGNS AND SYMPTOMS

Insect stings
- Painful, itching, rash-like lesion at the sting site
- Swelling and reddening
- Systemic allergic reaction with a combination of shock; skin (rash, swelling, itching) symptoms; gastrointestinal symptoms; and respiratory symptoms

Spider bites
- Local reaction: pain, reddening, swelling, and itching
- Tissue death: A bright red mark appears within a few hours of the bite and can evolve within 48 to 72 hours into a blood blister surrounded by purple discoloration or blanching. A purple lesion develops, forming an ulcer that can take weeks to months to heal.
- Systemic reaction of black widow bites: muscle cramping, hypertension, increased heart rate, profuse sweating, salivation, tearing, fluid in airway, abdominal rigidity, chest tightness, nausea, and vomiting. Death in young children is as high as 50% and results from cardiovascular collapse.

Snakebites
Crotalidae (pit viper) bites
- Intense local pain and burning, followed by swelling and numbness around the mouth that extends to the scalp
- Local bruising and blisters appear within the first few hours.
- Tissue death extending throughout the bitten extremity generally ensues without treatment.
- Nausea, vomiting, weakness, chills, and sweating can also occur.
- Within several hours, neuromuscular involvement can develop (double vision, difficulty swallowing, lethargy, etc.).
- The dramatic and life-threatening effects are shock and neuromuscular dysfunction.

Elapidae (Coral Snake) Bites
- Characterized by mild local signs and symptoms (pain, swelling), but significant neurologic effects that include loss of sensation in the bitten extremity, numbness or tingling, weakness, muscle spasm or cramps, and paralysis

CAUSES

Contact with animal or insect

SCOPE

See Description

 Diagnosis

QUESTIONS THE DOCTOR MAY ASK

N/A

WHAT THE DOCTOR LOOKS FOR

- Infection
- Tissue damage
- Nerve damage (loss of muscle power, sensory deficits)
- Rarely, skull fracture, major vessel injury, abdominal penetration, and chest trauma

Animal bite
- History-taking should include the type of animal, the apparent health of the animal and any provocation for the attack, the location of the bite, the rabies immunization status of the animal, and the tetanus immunization status of the child.

Insect and spider bites
- A description of the offender is important (particularly spiders). The black widow, about the size of a quarter, is glossy black, gray, or brown with a red, orange, or yellow hourglass-shaped marking on the bottom of the abdomen. The brown recluse spider is small (1–1.5 centimeters), with a brown violin-shaped mark on the back

Snakebites
- Pit vipers have a pit just in front of the eye, fangs, elliptical or slit-like pupil, somewhat triangular shape to the head, rattles (at times)
- Coral snakes are red, yellow, and black striped (specifically, red stripes bordered by yellow stripes) snakes. They have round pupils and rows of small teeth.
- Nonpoisonous snakes also have round pupils, rows of small teeth, no pit, and a double row of subcaudal plates.
- All snakebite wounds should be inspected for fang punctures. When present, the distance between them should be measured.

TESTS AND PROCEDURES

Blood tests, urinalysis

Animal Bites and Stings

 Treatment

GENERAL MEASURES

Animal bites
- Provide emergency first aid as needed, including control of bleeding
- Copious washing of the wound
- Closure of wounds, often by suturing
- Because of the risk of infection, hand wounds probably should not be sutured.

Insect stings
- If the stinger remains in the skin, it should be removed by flicking or scraping with a fingernail.
- Mild reactions can be treated with ice or cold compresses. Moderate reactions may require an antihistamine such as diphenhydramine orally for several days. Mild or severe anaphylactic reactions require epinephrine.

Brown recluse spider bites
- Mild bites: Frequent cleaning with soap and water, ice compresses initially, immobilization and elevation, use of diphenhydramine for itching, and an analgesic may also be considered.
- Large areas of tissue death may require surgery

Snakebites
- Rapid transport to medical facility, removal of jewelry/clothing from affected extremity, immobilization of the area.
- If possible, the snake should be killed and brought in for identification. The head of a dead snake must be handled with care since it can deliver a venomous bite for up to 1 hour after death/decapitation.

ACTIVITY

N/A

DIET

N/A

Medications

COMMONLY PRESCRIBED DRUGS

- Antibiotics are indicated for wounds with obvious infection and wounds at high risk for becoming infected, such as deep punctures, cat bites, and wounds involving the face or hands.
- Amoxicillin and clavulanic acid (Augmentin), or penicillin
- Rabies prevention is recommended for bites by bats; skunks; raccoons; foxes; coyotes; and unknown, unobservable dogs and cats. It is not recommended following bites by observable healthy dogs and cats or most rodents or rabbits. Human rabies immune globulin (RIG), human diploid cell rabies vaccine (HDCV), or rabies vaccine adsorbed (RVA) may be given.
- Tetanus immune globulin
- Snakebite antivenom

 ## Follow-Up

WHAT TO EXPECT

- Animal bites
  Fortunately, most injury from animal bites is trivial, but infections are not uncommon, and fatalities do occur rarely.
- Insect and spider bites
  Most bites do not produce serious effects; some bites can cause severe local and systemic reactions, including death. The most severe reactions and the rare fatalities occur with greater frequency in children.
- Snakebites
  Because only 15% of all snake bites are from poisonous snakes, and only about two-thirds of those involve true envenomation, the majority of bites cause only local injury.

PREVENTION

N/A

 ## Common Questions and Answers

Q: Which are the dangerous spiders?
A: Black, red, and brown widow spiders.

Q: What is the first aid for bites?
A: Wash thoroughly with saline.

Q: What is first aid for mild insect bites?
A: Ice.

Anorexia

 ## Basics

DEFINITION

Anorexia is an illness characterized by the refusal to eat, with resulting weight loss or failure to gain weight. The person with anorexia has an intense fear of gaining weight or becoming fat, and may have a misperception of body size. Females may stop menstruating. The person may regularly engage in binge eating or purging.

Mild
- Mildly distorted body image
- Weight more than 90% of average weight for height
- No symptoms or signs of excess weight loss
- Healthy weight loss methods (more than 1000 calories/day, moderate exercise, no purging)

Moderate
- Moderate distortion of body image unchanged with weight loss
- Weight less than 90% of average weight for height with refusal to stop further weight loss
- Symptoms or signs of weight loss associated with denial of any problem existing
- Unhealthy means to lose weight (less than 1000 calories/day, excessive exercise or purging)

Severe
- Grossly distorted body image unchanged with weight loss
- Weight 85% of average weight for height with refusal to stop further weight loss
- Symptoms or signs of extreme malnutrition, often coexisting with denial regarding thinness
- Unhealthy means of losing weight (less than 1000 calories/day, excessive exercise or purging)

SIGNS AND SYMPTOMS

- Eating habits, rituals, behavior
- Distorted body image
- Use of laxatives, diet pills, diuretics, emetics
- Presence of binge or purge behavior
- Absence of regular menstrual cycles
- Excessive exercise
- Weakness and fatigue
- Cold intolerance
- Headaches
- Abdominal pain
- Irregular bowel habits
- Mood disorder
- Anxiety
- Personality disorder
- Substance abuse
- Suicidal tendencies
- Yellowish complexion
- Low blood pressure
- Slow heart rate
- Low body temperature
- Weight 15% below ideal
- Short stature
- Degree of emaciation
- Dry skin
- Swelling

CAUSES

A combination of biologic, psychologic, and social factors. Risk factors include:
- A culture that equates thinness with beauty and happiness
- Families that are achievement-oriented, intrusive, enmeshed, unable to resolve conflicts, and who are overinvested in food, diet, weight, appearance, or physical fitness
- Being female with low self-esteem and having conflicts and doubts about identity or autonomy

SCOPE

Generally adolescent and young adult women

Diagnosis

QUESTIONS THE DOCTOR MAY ASK

- How do you feel about yourself?
- What made you start dieting?
- How do you handle weight control?
- How much do you want to weigh?
- How often do you weigh yourself?
- Do you vomit or use laxatives?
- How often and how much are you exercising?

WHAT THE DOCTOR LOOKS FOR

- Signs and symptoms of anorexia
- Complications, including:
  - ▶ Hormone imbalance
  - ▶ Cardiac disturbances
  - ▶ Gastrointestinal disorders
  - ▶ Neurologic disorder (weakness, nerve disorder, altered body temperature)
  - ▶ Cognitive (impaired concentration and alertness, distractibility, apathy, sleeping problems)
  - ▶ Gynecologic (absence of menstruation)
  - ▶ Musculoskeletal disorders
  - ▶ Dental (tooth erosion, salivary gland enlargement)
- Associated illnesses (depression, suicidal tendencies, sexual abuse)

TESTS AND PROCEDURES

- Blood tests
- Urinalysis
- Stool sample
- Electrocardiogram (EKG)
- Chest X-ray
- Upper gastrointestinal series (optional)
- Barium enema (optional)

 ## Treatment

GENERAL MEASURES

- A multidisciplinary approach is needed to make the diagnosis of anorexia nervosa. Evaluation should include a psychotherapist and a nutritionist.
- Hospitalization may be required.
- Weight gain should occur gradually over several weeks.
- Therapy lasts several years.

ACTIVITY

N/A

DIET

- Malnourished adolescents with anorexia nervosa have a lowered rate of metabolism, and initial energy requirements may be as low as 800–1000 calories/day.
- Calorie intake should be increased by 200–300 calories every 2–3 days as tolerated.
- Expected rate of weight gain varies, but a rate of 0.36 pounds/day has been shown to be safe in adolescents with anorexia nervosa.

Anorexia

 ## Medications

COMMONLY PRESCRIBED DRUGS

- Estrogen and calcium replacement for prevention of osteoporosis
- Stool softeners for constipation; avoid laxatives
- Antidepressants for depression
- Intravenous fluids may be required.

 ## Follow-Up

WHAT TO EXPECT

- 50% have good outcome, 25% have intermediate outcome, and 25% do poorly.
- Of those with satisfactory outcome, one-third recover by 3 years, one-third recover by 6 years, and one-third recover by 12 years.

Good outcome for those with:
- High educational achievement
- Early age of onset
- Good emotional adjustment
- Improvement in body image after weight gain
- Good initial ego strength
- Supportive family

Poor outcome for those with:
- Late age of onset
- Continued distortion of body image
- Pre-illness obesity
- Vomiting or laxative abuse
- Marked depression, obsessive behavior
- Family dysfunction
- Male gender

SIGNS TO WATCH

Signs that indicate problems include:
- Weight loss or failure to gain weight after institution of dietary program
- Salt imbalances
- Willful behavior and acting out
- Increased depression or mood disturbance

Emergency hospitalization may be required for:
- Low blood pressure
- Hypothermia (temperature, 36°C)
- Salt (electrolyte) imbalance
- Heart rate less than 55 beats/minute
- Gray-out (a fuzzy light-headed feeling) or fainting
- Weight below 75% ideal
- Uncontrollable binging and purging
- Acute food refusal
- Persistent weight loss
- Dehydration
- Acute psychiatric emergencies
- Medical complication of malnutrition (e.g., seizures, heart failure)
- Other conditions

PREVENTION

N/A

 ## Common Questions and Answers

Q: Should those without menstrual cycles be started on hormonal replacement?
A: Yes, adolescents should begin hormone therapy. Oral contraceptive pills are easiest to use. Often the patient does not wish to take hormones because he or she is fearful of weight gain.

Q: Should the patient be allowed to exercise as an outpatient?
A: Exercise should be restricted until the patient's weight has improved. Exercise often can be used as a bargaining tool in the behavioral management of these patients. If the patient maintains a minimum of 91% ideal body weight, he or she may exercise. If the weight decreases, exercise is again restricted.

Apnea

 Basics

DESCRIPTION

Apnea is a breathing disorder characterized by cessation of airflow lasting more than 20 seconds. In central apnea, air stops flowing because the drive to breathe is absent from the central nervous system. In obstructive apnea, the respiratory drive is present but the airway is blocked. The most common complications are low levels of oxygen in the blood, high levels of carbon dioxide, and a slow heart rate. If low oxygen levels are severe or persistent, damage to the heart, lungs, and other organ systems may result.

- Apparent life-threatening events (ALTE) refer to apneic events that to the child's caretaker appear life-threatening.
- Less than 10% of infants who die of sudden infant death syndrome (SIDS) had an ALTE before their death (SIDS by definition gives no warning).
- Apnea in full-term infants is most often caused by gastroesophageal reflux (GER).

SIGNS AND SYMPTOMS

Periods without breathing lasting more than 20 seconds

CAUSES

- Prematurity, immature respiratory control
- Infection
- Gastrointestinal reflux (GER)
- Neurologic disorders (asphyxia, seizure, central nervous system disorders)
- Pharmacologic (accidental drug ingestion, alcohol, poisoning)
- Metabolic (low blood sugar, low oxygen in blood, overheating)
- Cardiac (irregular heart rhythm, congenital heart disease)
- Anemia
- Inherited disorders
- Behavioral (breath-holding spells, excitement or agitation)
- Anatomic (enlarged tonsils or adenoids, obesity, foreign body, oral or craniofacial mal-formations)

SCOPE

- Some periodic apnea normally occurs in all infants.
- The amount and duration of apnea are related to maturity and age of the infant.
- Over 50% of premature infants develop apnea.
- Premature infants usually outgrow their apnea when they reach term age.
- Some infants may exhibit apnea of over 20 seconds in duration without apparent adverse effects.

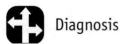 Diagnosis

QUESTIONS THE DOCTOR MAY ASK

- Was the baby moving his or her chest with or without evidence of airflow?
- Was the child awake or asleep when the event occurred?
- Was there a color change (pale, cyanotic, red)?
- Was there a change in the child's muscle tone (floppy versus stiff)?
- Was the episode related to feeding or preceded by coughing, choking, gagging, vomiting, or crying?
- Was there a change in the child's mental status during or after the event?
- Was there any urinary or stool incontinence during the event?
- Has there been a change in the child's school performance?
- Does the child have headaches or daytime sleepiness?

WHAT THE DOCTOR LOOKS FOR

- Apnea
- Periodic breathing
- Snoring
- Central breathing syndrome
- Breath-holding spells
- Airway obstruction or deformities
- Many times, the patient is in excellent health before the apneic event.
- Assessment of health before the apneic event:
  ▶ Evidence of infection (e.g., fever, rhinorrhea, nasal congestion, cough, diarrhea)
  ▶ Gestational age (full-term or premature)
  ▶ History of seizures or gastroesophageal reflux
  ▶ Snoring (snoring is never normal in a child)

TESTS AND PROCEDURES

- Blood tests
- Sleep study (polysomnography)
- X-ray of chest, neck, and head, milk scan
- Computed tomography (CT) scan or magnetic resonance imaging (MRI) of head (optional)
- Home studies are now available.
  - Advantage: study done in the child's usual environment
  - Disadvantages: no monitoring for problems, no technical support if problems arise

Apnea

 Treatment

GENERAL MEASURES

- Antireflux therapy:
  - Thickened feedings (add 1–3 teaspoons of rice cereal per ounce of formula)
  - Positioning (prone position for sleeping)
  - Medication
- Surgical removal of tonsils or adenoids may be required.

DIET

Weight loss is treatment for obesity-related obstructive sleep apnea.

ACTIVITY

N/A

 Medications

COMMONLY PRESCRIBED DRUGS

- Stimulants: caffeine, theophylline
- Supplemental oxygen and mechanical ventilation may be needed.
- Antireflux therapy: Reglan, Cisapride

Follow-Up

WHAT TO EXPECT

- Outcome depends on underlying cause of apnea.
- In premature infants, the outcome is excellent; premature infants usually outgrow apnea of prematurity by term to 4 weeks of age.
- In obstructive apnea caused by enlarged tonsils/adenoids, symptoms improve soon after surgery.
- In obese patients, outcome is variable because of difficulty in obtaining and maintaining weight loss.
- If using a home monitor, expect false alarms (stick-on electrodes have fewer false-positive alarms than do electrodes attached to wrap-around belts).

SIGNS TO WATCH

N/A

PREVENTION

Home apnea monitors
- Use is controversial.
- Monitoring technology now allows for the storing of information on a microchip, which can be downloaded for the physician to review.
- Do not prevent SIDS

 Common Questions and Answers

Q: When can monitoring be discontinued?
A: The decision to discontinue monitoring depends on the underlying reason for monitoring. When the infant is no longer thought to be at increased risk of cardiorespiratory arrest or sudden death or when the infant has tolerated at least one respiratory infection without significant events, monitoring may be discontinued. Medicolegal issues also affect the decision to discontinue monitoring.

Q: Does monitoring prevent SIDS?
A: Monitoring can prevent death from other causes, but it has not been shown to decrease the incidence of SIDS.

Q: When should medications for gastroesophageal reflux be discontinued?
A: Reevaluate the patient after 3 to 6 months of therapy. Discontinue the medications if the patient remains asymptomatic.

Appendicitis

 Basics

DEFINITION

Appendicitis is an acute inflammation of the appendix. If appendicitis is not recognized and treated (with surgical removal), the appendix may burst (perforate). Perforation of the appendix can cause inflammation of the abdominal lining, peritonitis, and lead to abscess formation.

SIGNS AND SYMPTOMS

- Vomiting
- Loss of appetite
- Low-grade fever (not over 102°F)
- Crampy abdominal pain that migrates to right lower quadrant
- Nausea, anorexia
- Patient prefers to lie still
- Diarrhea
- Change in bowel habits

CAUSE

N/A

SCOPE

- Usually occurs in children over 2 years old
- Peak incidence in teens and young adults
- Familial tendency toward appendicitis

 Diagnosis

QUESTIONS THE DOCTOR MAY ASK

Was car ride painful, e.g., going over bumps?
Interest in food? (should not be interested in eating)
Change in bowel (is it hard?)

WHAT THE DOCTOR LOOKS FOR

- Pain may start in mid-abdomen but move to right lower quadrant
- Breathing problems
- Pain in abdomen when hand on abdomen is released
- Guarding—not allowing deep palpation
- Rectal examination to localize tenderness to left side
- Listen to chest—pneumonia may cause right lower quadrant pain
- Sore throat—mesenteric adenitis may cause right lower quadrant pain
- Pain may be elicited by asking patient to cough or to hop on right foot.

TESTS AND PROCEDURES

- Blood tests—may perform several CBCs (complete blood cell counts)
- Abdominal X-ray
- Barium enema
- Ultrasound

 Treatment

GENERAL MEASURES

- Intravenous (IV) fluids
- Surgical consult
- Emergency appendectomy (removal of appendix)

DIET

N/A

ACTIVITY

N/A

Medications

COMMONLY PRESCRIBED DRUGS

None. Antibiotics for abscess.

 Follow-Up

WHAT TO EXPECT

• Recovery is rapid in children.
• Outcome is excellent without perforation, very good with perforation.

SIGNS TO WATCH

N/A

PREVENTION

N/A

 Common Questions and Answers

Q: Is appendicitis genetically inherited?
A: Appendicitis does show a tendency to occur among family members, but there is no definitive inheritance pattern.

Arthritis, Infectious

 Basics

DESCRIPTION

Infectious arthritis is an inflammation of a joint in response to the presence of infectious organisms.

SIGNS AND SYMPTOMS

- Pain
  - Worsens over 1 to 3 days
  - Does not wax and wane
- Fever occurs within first few days of illness in 75% of patients, less commonly in infants.
- Children usually appear ill.
- The joint appears warm and swollen.
- Decreased range of motion

CAUSES

Bacterial infection

SCOPE

- Predominant age: 2–6 years, adolescent
- Twice as common in males
- Predominantly affected joints: knee, hip, elbow, ankle

 Diagnosis

QUESTIONS THE DOCTOR MAY ASK

When did it start? Any Trauma? Medication? Other sites of infection?

WHAT THE DOCTOR LOOKS FOR

- Pain on movement of joint
- Red joint
- Swollen joint
- Other sites of infection on skin
- Trauma to joint area
- Puncture wounds

TESTS AND PROCEDURES

- Analysis of synovial fluids from joint
- Blood tests, blood culture
- X-rays
- Technetium-99 bone scan
- Ultrasound

Treatment

GENERAL MEASURES

- Drainage of infection should be done as soon as possible if bacterial cause is suspected.
- Antibiotic administration as soon as possible
- Immobilization of extremity
- Pain management

ACTIVITY

Rest the involved joint

DIET

N/A

 ## Medications

COMMONLY PRESCRIBED DRUGS

- Ampicillin
- Gentamicin
- Cefuroxime
- Chloramphenicol
- Cefazolin
- Clindamycin
- Ceftriaxone
- Penicillin
- Cefazolin

 ## Follow-Up

WHAT TO EXPECT

With appropriate antibacterial therapy, symptoms should improve within 2 days of initial drug administration.

SIGNS TO WATCH

Continued pain, fever, or lack of improvement in range of motion after 3 to 4 days of appropriate antibiotic treatment

PREVENTION

N/A

 ## Common Questions and Answers

Q: Will this infection cause permanent damage?
A: It may, depending on how much damage is done to the joint cartilage or bone.

Arthritis, Juvenile Rheumatoid

 Basics

DESCRIPTION

Juvenile rheumatoid arthritis (JRA) is a chronic inflammation of unknown cause in at least one joint that lasts for at least 6 weeks. Age of onset must be less than 16 years old. It can be subdivided into three major types:
- Pauciarticular: affects less than 5 joints
- Polyarticular: affects 5 or more joints and can occur at any age
- Systemic: characterized by high fevers and a pink rash. These children may also have enlarged lymph nodes, enlarged liver and spleen, and inflammation of the heart or lungs. The arthritis may not appear until weeks to months after the onset of the systemic symptoms. Systemic JRA can occur at any age.

SIGNS AND SYMPTOMS

- Arthritis in at least one joint
- Pain, inflammation
- Restricted range of motion in the affected joints
- Deformity of the affected joint
- Morning stiffness that improves after a hot shower/bath or with stretching and mild exercise is common in JRA.
- The joints often become sore/painful again in the late afternoon or evening.
- Patients with JRA generally do not report severe pain.
- May have eye pain, redness
- Enlarged spleen
- Skin rash—salmon color

CAUSES

Unknown, but genetics, autoimmunity, infection, and trauma may all play a role.

SCOPE

- JRA affects approximately 70,000 children in the United States.
- Affects girls twice as often as it affects boys, but one type usually affects boys
- Approximately 50% of children with JRA have the pauciarticular type.
- 40% have the polyarticular type.
- 10% have systemic-onset JRA.

 Diagnosis

QUESTIONS THE DOCTOR MAY ASK

Which joints?
How quickly is pain resolved by aspirin or other medicine?
Eye problems?
Skin rash?
Time of day of pain?

WHAT THE DOCTOR LOOKS FOR

The signs and symptoms of juvenile rheumatoid arthritis
Worn joints, skin rash, eye disease, enlarged spleen

TESTS AND PROCEDURES

- Blood tests
- X-rays

Treatment

GENERAL MEASURES

- Medication
- Physical and occupational therapy

ACTIVITY

Physical and occupational therapy are important in the management of JRA. The goal is to maintain range of motion, muscle strength, and function.

DIET

Maintain adequate calcium intake.

Medications

COMMONLY PRESCRIBED DRUGS

- Nonsteroidal antiinflammatory drugs (NSAIDS)
- Hydroxychloroquine
- Sulfasalazine
- Methotrexate
- Glucocorticoids

Follow-Up

WHAT TO EXPECT

- Responses to treatments for JRA vary tremendously.
  - Some patients may respond to NSAIDS within a week or two.
  - Others take 4–6 weeks to improve, or they may not respond at all.
  - Steroids usually start to relieve symptoms within a few days.
  - Hydroxychloroquine can take 4–8 weeks until the maximum benefit is seen.
- The waxing and waning nature of JRA itself adds to the variability of patients' responses to treatments.
- Outcome varies considerably.

SIGNS TO WATCH

- Eye pain or decrease in vision
- Muscle weakness or loss of muscle function
- Joint contractures

PREVENTION

N/A

Common Questions and Answers

Q: Will the patient outgrow JRA?
A: In some studies, up to 50% of patients with JRA still had active disease 10 years after diagnosis. Only 15%, however, had any loss of function.

Q: Will siblings of patients with JRA develop the disease?
A: Rarely, but it can occur.

Asthma

 Basics

DESCRIPTION

Asthma is the most common chronic illness in children. It is characterized by reversible airway obstruction, airway inflammation, and airway hyper-reactivity to a variety of stimuli.

SIGNS AND SYMPTOMS

- Coughing
- Wheezing
- Shortness of breath
- Chest tightness
- Triggers:
  - Infections (upper respiratory, sinusitis)
  - Allergies to dust mites, dander, pollen, mold
  - Cold air/weather changes
  - Exercise
  - Environmental triggers, e.g., cigarette smoke, strong odors, pollutants
  - Emotional factors, e.g., laughing, crying, fear
  - Drugs, including aspirin, nonsteroidal anti-inflammatory drugs (NSAIDS), beta blockers, ACE inhibitors
  - Food additives
  - Endocrine factors, e.g., menstruation, pregnancy, thyroid dysfunction

CAUSES

- Immune and inflammatory responses in the airways triggered by inhalation of an array of environmental allergens and infectious antigens
- Hereditary factors play a role.
- Allergies play a role.
- Viral infections during infancy are associated with the development of asthma.
- Exposure to cigarette smoke and other fumes or chemicals is associated with asthma.

SCOPE

- Recent increases in asthma prevalence, illness, and deaths
- Death rate of asthma among children rose over 30% between 1980 and 1987.
- Wheezing in children is extremely common in the industrialized world.
- Most episodes occur during viral infections.
- Most children outgrow their wheeze by age 6 years.
- 5–7% of all children (30–40% of those who wheeze) continue to wheeze, and asthma develops.
- Asthma is more common in boys than in girls up to age 10 years, but incidence is equal thereafter.

Diagnosis

QUESTIONS THE DOCTOR MAY ASK

- Is the patient compliant in taking his or her medications?
- Exercise tolerance?
- Association with infection?
- Do any household members smoke?
- How long does it take for the medicine to work?

WHAT THE DOCTOR LOOKS FOR

- Pattern of symptoms
- Home environment: heating system/air conditioning, fireplace, carpeting, pets, stuffed animals, cigarette smoking
- Physical examination

TESTS AND PROCEDURES

- Pulmonary function tests
- Allergy testing
- Blood tests
- Gastroesophageal reflux testing
- Bronchoscopy
- Chest, sinus X-rays

 Treatment

GENERAL MEASURES

- The first step in managing asthma is to educate the patient and his or her family about avoiding known triggers.
- Avoid airborne irritants (tobacco smoke, wood stoves, noxious fumes).
- Minimize dust-mite exposure:
  - ▸ Remove carpets (if possible) or use 3% tannic acid solution or benzyl benzoate for cleaning.
  - ▸ Put a plastic (vinyl) cover on mattresses and box spring.
  - ▸ Wash pillows, blankets, and sheets in hot water.

Asthma

- Avoid molds by decreasing relative humidity with a dehumidifier to 50%.
- Remove pets (if necessary).
- The child may be given a peak-flow meter to keep track of lung function at home.
  - The peak-flow meter measures the lungs' peak-flow rate (PEFR).
  - It is useful in treating patients with difficult-to-control asthma.
  - Dips in peak-flow rate precede onset of clinical asthmatic symptoms.
  - PEFR should be done at least once a day.
  - Specific medication guidelines depending on the PEFR should be individualized for each patient.

ACTIVITY

N/A

DIET

- Avoid foods or food additives (if truly allergic).
- Food-induced asthma is uncommon.

 Medications

COMMONLY PRESCRIBED DRUGS

- A variety of drugs are available to treat asthma. The type and combination of drugs should be individualized for each patient.
- Albuterol (Ventolin, Proventil)
- Terbutaline (Brethaire, Brethine)
- Metaproterenol (Alupent)
- Salmeterol (Serevent)
- Theophylline
- Nebulized atropine
- Ipratropium bromide (Atrovent)
- Cromolyn sodium (Intal)
- Nedocromil sodium (Tilade)
- Beclomethasone (Beclovent, Vanceril)
- Triamcinolone (Azmacort)
- Flunisolide (AeroBid)
- Prednisone
- Solu-medrol
- Troleandomycin (Tao)
- Helium: may improve airflow in severe asthma
- Routes of drug administration:
  - Inhaled (most effective): nebulizer
  - Metered-dose inhaler (MDI): Spinhaler
  - Oral (least effective; most side effects)

Asthma

 ## Follow-Up

WHAT TO EXPECT

- In acute asthma attacks, with appropriate therapy, improvement is usually seen within 24 to 48 hours.
- In chronic asthma, control of symptoms usually can be obtained within 1 month.
- With proper therapy and good compliance, the outcome is excellent.
- Complications include illness and death.
- Illness from asthma is characterized by:
  - Frequent hospitalizations and absence from school
  - Chronic symptoms affect activity level and function
  - Psychologic impact of having a chronic illness
  - Chronic recurrent atelectasis may lead to the development of localized bronchiectasis.
- The death rate from asthma is increasing. Currently, it is not known why the death rate has increased. In addition, there has been an increase in the number of life-threatening asthma attacks.

SIGNS TO WATCH FOR

- Decrease in peak-flow rate
- Increasing use of inhaled bronchodilators
- Subject not improving on enhanced home therapy

PREVENTION

- Comply with treatment regimen.
- Avoid known triggers of asthma attack.

 ## Common Questions and Answers

Q: Will my child outgrow his or her asthma?
A: Family history and allergies affect the ultimate outcome. Wheezing during the first 3 years of life is extremely common, with 40 to 50% of all children wheezing at some time. Many of these children do not develop asthma and outgrow their illness by school age. Some patients develop asthma again as young adults.

Q: Can my child become dependent on asthma medications?
A: Children do not become dependent on these medications as they would with narcotic agents. Daily asthma medications are required to maintain airway patency and to control airway inflammation.

Q: Will my child be on medications for the rest of his or her life?
A: This depends on the severity of the asthma. The types, doses, and frequency of asthma medications change over a patient's lifetime.

Q: Do inhaled steroids affect patient growth?
A: There is no convincing evidence of long-term growth suppression or bone demineralization in school-aged children. Further studies are in progress.

Ataxia

 ## Basics

DESCRIPTION

Ataxia is characterized by shaking movements of extremities, trunk, tongue, or eyes. Acute cerebellar ataxia after a benign viral infection is common in children, producing difficulty walking and moving. There are other forms of ataxia as well. Chronic ataxia usually signals a serious underlying disease (tumor, hereditary, or metabolic disorder).

SIGNS AND SYMPTOMS

- Tremor
- Difficulty walking
- Difficulty moving
- Incoordination
- Sensory disturbances
- Rhythmical oscillation of the eyes

CAUSES

- Consequence of infection
- Hereditary disorder
- Nervous system disorder
- Drug/alcohol ingestion
- Poisoning

SCOPE

The scope of ataxia depends on the cause.

 ## Diagnosis

QUESTIONS THE DOCTOR MAY ASK

- Onset
- Exposure to chickenpox
- Medication
- Ingestion of poison
- Change in personality
- Family history

WHAT THE DOCTOR LOOKS FOR

- Acute versus chronic ataxia
- Cause of ataxia
- Neurologic examination

TESTS AND PROCEDURES

- Toxicologic screen
- X-rays, magnetic resonance imaging (MRI), computed tomography (CT)
- Spinal tap
- Electroencephalogram (EEG)
- Blood tests
- Urinalysis

 ## Treatment

GENERAL MEASURES

Therapy as needed for any underlying condition.

ACTIVITY

N/A

DIET

N/A

Medications

COMMONLY PRESCRIBED DRUGS

- Steroids (prednisolone)
- Immunotherapy
- Acetazolamide

 ## Follow-Up

WHAT TO EXPECT

Acute postinfection ataxia usually resolves over days to weeks.

SIGNS TO WATCH

Persistence or worsening of symptoms

PREVENTION

N/A

 ## Common Questions and Answers

Q: What intoxications are most likely to cause ataxia?
A: Benzodiazepines, major anticonvulsants, alcohol, tricyclics, antihistamines, and others.

Q: How long can postinfectious ataxia last?
A: Rarely, it may last for months, but it should be improving during that time.

Q: What is the role of physical therapy for ataxia?
A: Physical therapy for ataxia is of limited value.

Attention Deficit Hyperactivity Disorder

 ## Basics

DESCRIPTION

Attention deficit hyperactivity disorder (ADHD) is characterized by persistent and inappropriate levels of inattention and/or hyperactivity-impulsivity.

SIGNS AND SYMPTOMS

- Fidgeting
- Difficulty remaining seated
- Easily distracted
- Can't wait turn
- Blurts out answers before question is complete
- Difficulty following directions
- Difficulty sustaining attention
- Shifts from one uncompleted task to another
- Difficulty playing quietly
- Talks excessively
- Interrupts others
- Doesn't seem to be listening
- Loses things
- Engages in physically dangerous activities without considering consequences

CAUSES

The cause is not identified in most cases.

SCOPE

- Affects 3–5% of school-aged children
- Four times more frequent in males
- Affects adolescents and adults; prevalence in these populations unknown
- 30–40% of children with ADHD have at least one first-degree relative with ADHD.

 ## Diagnosis

QUESTIONS THE DOCTOR MAY ASK

- Does the child:
  - finish work, chores?
  - squirm or fidget?
  - lose or forget things needed for homework or other tasks?
  - interrupt games, questions, or conversations?
  - have difficulty waiting his/her turn?
- How does the child attend to activities at home/in school? (Discrepancy, especially if worse at home, suggests that other diagnoses should be considered.)
- Does the child's behavior differ for tasks versus play activities? (Many children with ADHD can pay attention during play activities, but not while performing tasks.)

WHAT THE DOCTOR LOOKS FOR

- History: impulsive behavior, distractability, level of activity, family history
- Description of behaviors (frequency, duration, intensity)
- Symptom onset (usually prior to age 7)
- Developmental, medical, family, and social history focusing on diseases in differential diagnoses
- Physical and neurologic examination is usually normal.

TESTS AND PROCEDURES

- Many rating scales to assess ADHD exist.
- Report from school
- Neurologic examination to exclude systemic disease (only rarely is a systemic disease found)

 ## Treatment

GENERAL MEASURES

Behavioral counseling and educational interventions are important components of treatment.

ACTIVITY

N/A

DIET

N/A

Attention Deficit Hyperactivity Disorder

 ## Medications

COMMONLY PRESCRIBED DRUGS

- Methylphenidate (Ritalin): Eighty percent of children with ADHD improve significantly; individual response is highly variable.
- Dextroamphetamine (Dexedrine)
- Pemoline (Cylert)
- Clonidine
- Tricyclic antidepressants

 ## Follow-Up

WHAT TO EXPECT

- Outcome is frequently good with prompt diagnosis and appropriate treatment.
- Assess school performance.
- Check for associated behavior problems.
- Assess family and peer relationships.
- Check for medication side effects every 4 to 6 months.
- Assess continuing need for medication yearly.

SIGNS TO WATCH FOR

- School failure (33% kept back a grade before reaching high school)
- Poor peer relationships
- Sleep problems (over 50%)
- Poor fine motor skills
- Increased risk of accidental injury
- Additional mental disorders (over 40%)
- Learning disabilities (30%)

PREVENTION

N/A

 ## Common Questions and Answers

Q: At what age can you begin to make the diagnosis of ADHD?
A: No lower age limit has been identified for ADHD. There are a wide range of normal activity levels and attention spans in preschool-aged children. Be cautious about making the diagnosis in a child under age 4 years.

Q: Should stimulant medication be prescribed on weekends and over the summer?
A: Family and peers of some children with ADHD benefit from continuous use; periods off medication ("vacations") may minimize the long-term effects on appetite and growth. Children engaged in school-like or school-related tasks during the summer or on weekends may need to be on medication for these activities.

Q: What is the significance of neurologic finding of "soft signs"?
A: Soft signs are minor signs in neurologic examinations, such as uncoordinated, rapid movements. They are not specific for ADHD.

Bell Palsy

 ## Basics

DESCRIPTION

Bell palsy is an acute paralysis of the face muscles, usually on one side.

SIGNS AND SYMPTOMS

- Pain (ear pain is common first symptom; paralysis follows rapidly)
- Difficulty closing eyes, drinking, and controlling salivation
- Loss of taste
- Numbness of face, neck, ear, or tongue
- Headache, malaise, muscle ache, sore throat
- Abnormally acute hearing
- Decreased tearing

CAUSES

- Unknown. Some causes are from trauma to ear region.
- Associated with viral illness.

SCOPE

- Over half of cases preceded by upper respiratory symptoms
- Incidence: 20 per 100,000 persons
- Incidence increases with each decade of life.
- Positive family history in 10%

 ## Diagnosis

QUESTIONS THE DOCTOR MAY ASK

- Ear pain?
- Tearing of eyes?
- Change in hearing?
- Trauma?
- Recent infection?

WHAT THE DOCTOR LOOKS FOR

- Time course of symptoms
- Birth history, birth trauma, history of other developmental defects or syndromes
- Trauma to ear area
- Previous history of palsy
- Family history
- Recent viral illness
- Physical examination
- Complete neurologic examination

TESTS AND PROCEDURES

- Blood tests
- Audiography and other ear testing
- Tear testing
- Electrodiagnostic tests
- Computed tomography (CT) or magnetic resonance imaging (MRI) of head

Treatment

GENERAL MEASURES

- Artificial tears during the day, bland eye ointment at night, dark glasses during the day, patching of eye if needed
- Muscle exercises

ACTIVITY

N/A

DIET

N/A

Medications

COMMONLY PRESCRIBED DRUGS

- Prednisone—must be used early in disease
- Acyclovir

Follow-Up

WHAT TO EXPECT

- Overall outcome is good; 60–80% of children have complete recovery.
- Impossible to predict who will progress to severe, complete paralysis
- 10% recurrence rate
- After recurrence, further recurrences more likely

SIGNS TO WATCH

Lack of improvement in expected time period. The majority of cases of Bell palsy resolve in 4 to 6 months, and all Bell palsy cases should resolve in 12 months.

PREVENTION

N/A

Common Questions and Answers

Q: Why are artificial tears needed?
A: Eyelids do not close, causing the eyes to become dried since eyelids help spread tears to keep eye moist.

Birthmarks

 ## Basics

DESCRIPTION

Birthmarks are colored lesions of the skin. There are four types of birthmarks: hemangiomas, salmon patches, vascular malformations, and brown patches (nevi).

SIGNS AND SYMPTOMS

- Raised, bright red-pink color, sharply demarcated border, stippled surface (strawberry birthmark)
- Raised, smooth, bluish mark
- Port-wine stains: apparent at birth, pink-to-red sharp-edged bump, possibly slightly raised, darkens with age
- Brown areas of irregular density

CAUSES

- Abnormal growth of blood vessels and skin tissue
- Increased brown pigment in skin

SCOPE

Birthmarks are common; some are apparent at birth, while others are not present until adolescence or adulthood.

 ## Diagnosis

QUESTIONS THE DOCTOR MAY ASK

- Growth of birthmark?
- Breeding?
- Change in color?

WHAT THE DOCTOR LOOKS FOR

Type, size, and number of birthmarks

TESTS AND PROCEDURES

- Rarely done
- X-rays
- Magnetic resonance imaging (MRI)

 ## Treatment

GENERAL MEASURES

- No therapy is indicated in more than 95% of strawberry birthmarks. They typically enlarge and then regress in about a year.
- For strawberry birthmark that bleeds: direct pressure
- For ulcerated strawberry birthmark: observation or wet compresses and topical antibacterial drugs
- Port wine stain: cosmetic camouflage or laser treatment

ACTIVITY

N/A

DIET

N/A

Medications

COMMONLY PRESCRIBED DRUGS

- Steroids
- Interferon

 ## Follow-Up

WHAT TO EXPECT

Outcome depends on the type and location of birthmarks.

SIGNS TO WATCH

- Ulceration
- Bleeding
- Infection
- Neurologic signs or symptoms

PREVENTION

N/A

 ## Common Questions and Answers

Q: What will happen to the strawberry birthmark on a child's wrist?
A: Expect it to enlarge, acquire a bluish hue, and then get smaller.

Q: What happens to the "stork bite" on the back of the neck?
A: It fades.

Q: What do you call the redness on eyelids or forehead?
A: Some call it Angel's kiss.

Bone Infection

 Basics

DESCRIPTION

Infection of the bone, or osteomyelitis, is usually caused by a bacterial infection.

SIGNS AND SYMPTOMS

- Sudden onset of bone or joint pain and fever
- Refusal to bear weight on or move the extremity that is involved
- Fever
- Tenderness over affected bone
- As the infection progresses, swelling, warmth, and reddening of the skin overlying the infection may be noted.

CAUSES

Bacterial infection: staph, strep, salmonella, pseudomonas.

SCOPE

Incidence of 0.016% per year

 Diagnosis

QUESTIONS THE DOCTOR MAY ASK

- Fever?
- Pain?
- Redness and swelling?
- Trauma?
- Difficulty walking?
- Limp?

WHAT THE DOCTOR LOOKS FOR

Signs and symptoms of bone infection: tenderness in bone, warm skin, redness

TESTS AND PROCEDURES

- Blood tests
- Blood culture
- Biopsy of infected bone
- X-rays
- Bone scan

 Treatment

GENERAL MEASURES

- Antibiotics
- Aspiration of infected needle
- Surgery may be necessary.

ACTIVITY

N/A

DIET

N/A

Medications

COMMONLY PRESCRIBED DRUGS

Antibiotics

 ## Follow-Up

WHAT TO EXPECT

Patients should be followed to ensure adequate treatment of infection and continued growth of the extremity involved.

SIGNS TO WATCH

N/A

PREVENTION

N/A

? Common Questions and Answers

Q: Will osteomyelitis cause permanent damage in the bone?
A: If the growth plate is not damaged and the infection is adequately treated, there should be no permanent effects of osteomyelitis. If the growth plate is damaged, however, the affected limb may not grow evenly, or at all, even after the infection is treated.

Brain Injury

 Basics

DESCRIPTION

Brain injury is damage to the brain sustained as a result of trauma, bleeding, or decreased blood flow to brain tissue. Manifestations may include loss of consciousness, seizures, fainting, and paralysis on one side of the body. Concussion is loss of consciousness at the time of impact. Head injury is frequently associated with trauma to the face, neck, or other parts of the body without permanent brain damage.

SIGNS AND SYMPTOMS

- Loss of consciousness
- Signs of injury: bleeding, bruising, fracture
- Blood or fluid in ear or nose
- Labored breathing
- Neurologic deficit
- Unequal pupils
- Amnesia

CAUSE

Intentional or unintentional trauma, bleeding, or decreased blood flow

SCOPE

- Incidence of general trauma is approximately 86 per 1000 persons, of which 50% is head trauma.
- In children less than 2 years old, falls are the most common cause of trauma.

 Diagnosis

QUESTIONS THE DOCTOR MAY ASK

- Eyewitness accounts
- Did the injury precede loss of consciousness or did the child collapse and then become unresponsive?
- Abnormal movement of arms or eyes?
- Vomiting?
- Loss of bladder and/or bowel control?

WHAT THE DOCTOR LOOKS FOR

- A history of previous concussions, seizures, and details of who was caring for the child
- Cause of fall or injury
- Complications
- Physical examination
- Neurologic examination
- Unequal pupils
- Spinal fluid in ears or nose

TESTS AND PROCEDURES

- X-rays
- Computed tomography (CT)
- Blood tests

Treatment

GENERAL MEASURES

- Provide first aid as needed.
- Do not move victim of a fall unless it is necessary to protect safety (burning building, etc.).
- Call 9-1-1.
- Victim needs prompt medical evaluation.
- Hospitalization is required.
- Surgery may be required.

ACTIVITY

N/A

DIET

N/A

 ## Medications

COMMONLY PRESCRIBED DRUGS

N/A

 ## Follow-Up

WHAT TO EXPECT

- Outcome depends on severity of injury.
- Neurologists, neurosurgeon, ophthalmologists, audiologists, psychologists, and physical therapists may be helpful.
- Approximately 2% of persons with severe head injury develop seizures.
- Patients who have sustained moderate to severe head injury often have academic difficulties, memory abnormalities, disinhibition, and other complications.
- Referral to multidisciplinary rehabilitation center may be beneficial.

SIGNS TO WATCH

Cognitive difficulties, hyperactivity, seizures, movement disorders, paralysis, visual/hearing disturbances, headache

PREVENTION

- Properly fitting helmets should be worn while riding a bicycle, roller-skating, and similar activities.
- Children should be properly restrained while riding in a car.

 ## Common Questions and Answers

Q: What are the specific signs of increased intracranial pressure?
A: Cushing's reflex in association with deterioration in mental status. Change in pupils or occular motility, or onset of posturing may also indicate increased ICP.

Q: Will a CT scan detect all skull fractures?
A: It does not always demonstrate fractures at the base of the skull.

Brain Tumor

 ## Basics

DESCRIPTION

A brain tumor is an abnormal growth of new tissue in the central nervous system. The tumor may be benign (noncancerous) or malignant (cancerous).

SIGNS AND SYMPTOMS

- Headache, particularly if it lasts more than 1 week if daily or 1 month if intermittent
- Vomiting, particularly if associated with headache and if it occurs in morning
- New onset of neurologic symptoms, such as double vision, visual field disturbances, weakness, incoordination, rhythmic oscillation of the eyes, or new onset seizures
- Changes in behavior or school performance

CAUSES

- No specific causative agents are known (diet, environmental exposure, etc.).

SCOPE

- Second most common cause of cancer in children
- Incidence is increasing.
- Highest risk is in infants, and decreases thereafter.
- Slight male predominance

 ## Diagnosis

QUESTIONS THE DOCTOR MAY ASK

- Change in personality, behavior, school performance?
- Early morning vomiting?
- Recent onset of seizures?
- Double vision?
- Headache?

WHAT THE DOCTOR LOOKS FOR

- Head circumference
- Neurologic examination
- Strength
- Coordination
- Eye movements
- Changes in mental status
- History of neurofibromatosis in patient or family, café-au-lait spots

TESTS AND PROCEDURES

- Magnetic resonance imaging (MRI)
- Computed tomography (CT)

 ## Treatment

GENERAL MEASURES

- Surgery
- Radiation therapy
- Chemotherapy

ACTIVITY

N/A

DIET

- As desired
- Loss of appetite or overeating (steroid-induced) can be a problem.

Medications

COMMONLY PRESCRIBED DRUGS

- Dexamethasone
- CCNU, vincristine, procarbazine
- Cisplatin, cyclophosphamide
- Carboplatin
- Drugs are most often used in combination.
- New protocols are always under development.

 ## Follow-Up

WHAT TO EXPECT

- Prognosis varies depending on tumor type and location.
- Patients must be monitored closely.
- Improvement often is evident after surgery.

SIGNS TO WATCH

- Loss of motor function
- Increased urination
- Vomiting
- Seizures

PREVENTION

N/A

 ## Common Questions and Answers

Q: Are my other children at risk for getting a brain tumor?
A: No.

Q: Did something I do cause this?
A: No. Furthermore, the claims made about high-power lines and cellular phones causing brain tumors or cancer are unproven.

Q: Is this inherited?
A: No, except for tumors associated with neurofibromatosis.

Breast-Feeding

Basics

DESCRIPTION

- The human breast makes colostrum toward the latter part of pregnancy and for 2 to 5 days after birth. Colostrum is high in protein and minerals, low in carbohydrates and fat. It also contains antibodies.
- Hormonal and physical stimuli are necessary for the mother's breasts to engorge with milk in the first week after birth.
- The regular, frequent, and complete emptying of breasts by infant is the physical stimulus for increasing production of milk.
- Breast milk supply diminishes when breasts are not emptied completely.

SIGNS AND SYMPTOMS

N/A

CAUSES

N/A

SCOPE

Greater incidence of breast-feeding seen with higher maternal education, socioeconomic status, and family support of breast-feeding.

Diagnosis

QUESTIONS THE DOCTOR MAY ASK

- Motivation for breast-feeding
- Planned length of breast-feeding
- Let down reflex—leakage of milk
- Adequate rest and nutrition
- Technique used in breast-feeding

WHAT THE DOCTOR LOOKS FOR

- The first several well-child-care visits are important to troubleshoot and help support continued breast-feeding.
- Frequency of feeds should be every 1.5–3 hours in the newborn period.
- Length of feeding sessions should be 10–20 minutes per breast.

- Maternal comfort with breast-feeding ensures the success of the infant latching onto the breast.
- The infant should appear to be satisfied feeding and have a normal infant sleep pattern.
- Infant urine output: After milk supply is in, infant should make 5–6 wet diapers per day minimum.
- Stool frequency: One stool per feed is typical in the newborn receiving adequate nourishment; however, frequency may vary to a low of 1 stool per week.
- Maternal diet and vitamin intake should be adequate to maintain nutritional needs.
- Older infant (8–12 months) shows signs of natural weaning.
- Clues to inadequate milk supply:
  - Scantily wet diapers, especially with pinkish tinge
  - Infrequent stools
  - Frequent feeding without apparent satisfaction or sleep after sessions
  - Jaundice
- Weight gain: Infants should return to birth weight or greater by 2 weeks of age (after an expected weight loss of 10% of initial birth weight).

TESTS AND PROCEDURES

- Rarely necessary

Treatment

GENERAL MEASURES

- Home-visit nurses, especially for first-time mothers, should visit the mother and infant for weight checks, assessments of hydration status, and assessment of breast-feeding technique.
- Nipple care for sore, cracked nipples:
  - Vary nursing positions frequently.
  - Expose nipples to air.
  - Allow breast milk to dry on nipples.
  - Avoid soap.
  - Avoid prolonged nursing sessions.
- Breast-feeding counselor or support group can be helpful.
- Avoid supplementing with formula in the first several weeks unless signs of dehydration

- Use milk-enhancement techniques as necessary:
  - ▶ Rest.
  - ▶ Increase maternal fluid intake.
  - ▶ Increase frequency of nursing.
  - ▶ Avoid formula supplements.
  - ▶ Gain reassurance through counseling and frequent weight checks of infant.

ACTIVITY

N/A

DIET

A nursing mother should pay particular attention to her diet and fluid intake by ensuring the following:
- Good nutrition supplemented by daily prenatal vitamins
- Calcium intake of at least 1200 milligrams/day
- Avoiding weight-reduction diets
- Increased caloric intake by 300 calories/day from baseline
- Fluid intake of 3 quarts per day
- Avoiding certain foods (berries, tomatoes, onions, broccoli, cabbage, chocolate, caffeine, and spicy foods) if infant has significant gas distress

 Medications

COMMONLY PRESCRIBED DRUGS

- Vitamin K intramuscular injection
- Iron
- Vitamin D

 Follow-Up

WHAT TO EXPECT

- Outcome of breast-feeding is excellent; nearly 100% of mothers should be able to breast-feed successfully.
- Early office visit and/or home visit is indicated for infants with early hospital discharge.
- Early phone contact for breast-feeding counseling
- Two-week visit to ensure adequate weight gain
- Severe maternal illness may interfere with breast-feeding.
- Maternal medication intake may interfere with breast-feeding.

SIGNS TO WATCH

- Inadequate infant weight gain
- Poor urine/stool output
- Lethargy
- Unsatisfied hunger
- Marked jaundice

PREVENTION

Maternal education (prenatal breast-feeding support classes), family support of nursing, and close follow-up is critical in preventing early failure of breast-feeding.

 Common Questions and Answers

Q: What are the advantages of breast-feeding?
A: Breast milk is the most natural form of nutrition and provides vital nutrients and antibodies to improve newborn health. Breast milk is the most efficiently digested infant food. Breast-feeding also enhances maternal-infant bonding.

Q: When can I start using a bottle so that I may go back to work or leave the baby with a sitter?
A: It is generally advisable to breast-feed exclusively for at least the first 3 weeks of life until the mother's milk supply is fairly well established and supply is meeting demand. After this time, the mother can tailor feeds to meet her lifestyle demands. Ideally, pumped breast milk can be stored and given to the baby by the father or a sitter, but many mothers are also able to maintain several nursing sessions a day successfully while supplementing with formula for the other feeds if weaning is done slowly and consistently. There is benefit to any breast milk that an infant gets, so a flexible supportive counseling attitude of the physician may prolong nursing even for the working mother.

Q: What drugs should be avoided by breast feeding women?
A: Alcohol, stimulants, narcotics, nicotine, radioactive material, aspirin, ergotamine, isoniazid, lithium.

Q: Which drugs have no effect?
A: Ampicillin, cephalosporin, and furosemide are a few.

Breath-Holding Attack

 ## Basics

DESCRIPTION

- A breath-holding attack is an involuntary event in which the child stops breathing.
- It may be associated with loss of consciousness and seizure activity.

SIGNS AND SYMPTOMS

Periods of suspended breathing

CAUSES

- Abnormality of nervous system regulation
- Abnormality in respiratory control
- Usually brought on by anger, frustration, fear, or minor injury

SCOPE

- Occurs in approximately 5% of children
- Onset between 6 months and 2 years of age
- Rare after 6 years of age

 ## Diagnosis

QUESTIONS THE DOCTOR MAY ASK

- Events that preceded attack?
- Did arms and legs move?
- Did the child wake up and resume activity or was he/she sleepy?
- How does the child handle frustration?

WHAT THE DOCTOR LOOKS FOR

- Preceding circumstances and parents' reaction to the event
- The results of a physical examination are normal, including the neurologic examination.

TESTS AND PROCEDURES

- Electroencephalogram (EEG)
- Electrocardiogram (EKG)

 ## Treatment

GENERAL MEASURES

- Reassurance: These spells do not harm the child. Normal breathing resumes after loss of consciousness.
- Attempts to give mouth-to-mouth resuscitation to children with breath-holding spells are unnecessary.

ACTIVITY

N/A

DIET

N/A

Medications

COMMONLY PRESCRIBED DRUGS

None

 ## Follow-Up

WHAT TO EXPECT

- Follow-up is based on the amount of support the parents need in learning to manage these spells.
- The parents may be referred to a mental health professional if they are unable to discipline child for fear of inducing breath-holding spells.
- The child may learn to trigger spells if the result is getting what he or she wants.

SIGNS TO WATCH

Call 9-1-1 if loss of consciousness is greater than 1 minute. Clear the mouth of food/foreign bodies during episode.

PREVENTION

Work with child to handle frustration

 ## Common Questions and Answers

Q: Are children with breath-holding spells more stubborn or disobedient than other children?
A: No. Recent studies have found no difference in the behavioral profiles of children who have breath-holding spells and children who do not have breath-holding spells.

Bronchiolitis

 ## Basics

DESCRIPTION

Bronchiolitis is an acute lower respiratory illness that causes obstruction of the small airways of the lung. It is characterized by rapid, noisy breathing.

SIGNS AND SYMPTOMS

- Runny nose with thick nasal secretions
- Cough
  ▶ Initially, hoarse cough for 3 to 5 days
  ▶ Progresses to deep, wet cough of increased frequency
- Poor feeding
- Dehydration
- Low-grade fever
- Restlessness or lethargy
- Cessation of breathing (seen in younger patients)
- Color change: bluish discoloration around eyes, lips, and nail beds (cyanosis)
- Respiratory distress

CAUSES

- Viral infection
- Direct contact with nasal secretions from an infected individual
- Spread in the air (called aerosol spread) is less common.

SCOPE

- Peaks during the winter and early spring
- Most children are infected in the first 3 years of life; 80% within the first 12 months.
- More common in infants with:
  ▶ Lower socioeconomic status
  ▶ Crowded living conditions
  ▶ Delayed immunizations
  ▶ Exposure to cigarette smoke
  ▶ Bottle-feeding versus breast-feeding
- More serious the younger the child (less than 6 months old)
- Rarely fatal in otherwise healthy infants
- Approximately half of infants with bronchiolitis develop wheezing.

 ## Diagnosis

QUESTIONS THE DOCTOR MAY ASK

- Exposure to ill people?
- Evidence of lethargy?
- Fluid intake?
- History of asthma in family?
- Irritability, cyanosis?

WHAT THE DOCTOR LOOKS FOR

- Physical examination: fever, air exchange, cyanosis of lips, retraction (space between ribs caves in during breathing), irritability, lethargy
- Pulmonary examination: degree of airway distress
- Pneumonia or other complications
- Highest risk of complications seen with:
  ▶ Congenital heart disease
  ▶ Lung disease
  ▶ Cystic fibrosis
  ▶ Prematurity
  ▶ Immune system disorders

TESTS AND PROCEDURES

- Blood tests
- Pulse oximetry to assess oxygenation
- Arterial blood gasses
- Rapid viral identification
- Viral culture
- Chest x-ray

 ## Treatment

GENERAL MEASURES

- Most cases are mild and can be treated at home.
- Only 1–5% of previously healthy children require hospitalization.
- Hospitalization should be considered for infants and young children who:
  ▶ Were born prematurely
  ▶ Appear ill or toxic
  ▶ Are less than 3 months of age
  ▶ Have decreased oxygen saturation
  ▶ Have an underlying disease

ACTIVITY

N/A

DIET

Fluid intake is important.

Medications

COMMONLY PRESCRIBED DRUGS

- None usually.
- Supplemental oxygen with humidity
- Bronchodilators
- Corticosteroids
- Antiviral agents (Ribavirin)
- RSV Hyperimmunoglobulin

 ## Follow-Up

WHAT TO EXPECT

- Most infants improve within 3 to 5 days.
- For most infants, the outcome is excellent.
- Illness and death are considerable in patients with an underlying chronic disease.
- 40–50% of infants have recurrent episodes of wheezing until 2 to 3 years of age:
  ▶ Some will develop asthma.
  ▶ Others have abnormal lung function later in childhood.

SIGNS TO WATCH

- Impending respiratory failure
- Sudden deterioration
- Fatigue may occur in infants who have prolonged and extensive disease.

 ## Common Questions and Answers

Q: How did my child get bronchiolitis?
A: Bronchiolitis is a common, seasonal, lower respiratory tract infection that is easily transmissible.

Q: Can my child become reinfected?
A: Children can become reinfected with bronchiolitis, and infection can occur more than once during the same respiratory season.

Q: Do patients with bronchiolitis need to be isolated?
A: Hospitalized patients who are virus-positive need to be isolated with other virus-positive patients and isolated from uninfected patients. Patients who are receiving ribavirin should be kept in isolation.

Q: Will my child develop asthma?
A: Significant numbers of infected children develop recurrent wheezing. Some eventually have asthma.

Campylobacter Infection

 ## Basics

DESCRIPTION

Campylobacter are a type of bacteria. The species of Campylobacter involved in human infections include *Campylobacter jejuni* (which causes enteritis), *Campylobacter fetus* (implicated in systemic illness), and *Campylobacter pylori* (a causative agent in gastritis). If the infection is not eradicated, a chronic phase results that can persist indefinitely.

SIGNS AND SYMPTOMS

- Colic
- Diarrhea (may be bloody)
- Fever
- Upper abdominal pain
- Bloating
- Nausea
- Vomiting
- Bad breath (halitosis)

CAUSES

Infection with campylobacter organism

SCOPE

- The number of Campylobacter infections equal and perhaps exceed the number of cases of inflammatory enteritis caused by other causes, with the highest attack rates observed in young children.
- 30–100% of chickens, turkeys, and water fowl are infected asymptomatically; swine, cattle, sheep, horses, rodents, and household pets (especially young pets) may also carry the organism. Contaminated water and milk sources also act as reservoirs for infections.

 ## Diagnosis

QUESTIONS THE DOCTOR MAY ASK

- Exposure to such children
- Diarrhea
- Vomiting
- Abdominal pain
- Exposure to unpasteurized milk products, well-water use, and inadequately cooked poulty
- Water supply

WHAT THE DOCTOR LOOKS FOR

- Exposure to unpasteurized milk products, well-water use, and inadequately cooked poultry
- Illness is characterized by fever, abdominal pain, and bloody diarrhea.
- The incubation period is 1–7 days and is usually self-limited by 5 to 7 days.
- *C. pylori* infection should be suspected in any patient with chronic abdominal pain.

TESTS AND PROCEDURES

- Stool culture
- Blood tests
- Culture of biopsy from stomach

 ## Treatment

GENERAL MEASURES

N/A

ACTIVITY

N/A

DIET

N/A

Medications

COMMONLY PRESCRIBED DRUGS

Antibiotics
- Erythromycin
- Ciprotoxacin
- Tetracycline
- Clindamycin
- Chorlamphenicol
- Ceftaxine

Follow-Up

WHAT TO EXPECT

- The prognosis is usually very good.
- Outcome can vary.
- If the infection is not eradicated, a chronic phase can persist for months.
- Once treated, symptoms should improve in 2 to 3 days.

SIGNS TO WATCH

N/A

PREVENTION

Thorough hand washing after contact with animals or animal products, proper cooling and storage of foods, pasteurization of milk, and chlorination of water supplies decreases the overall risk for infection.

Common Questions and Answers

Q: Are there any risks of Campylobacter infection to the pregnant patient?
A: Women infected symptomatically or asymptomatically may experience recurrent miscarriages or preterm deliveries. Life-threatening infections to the fetus or newborn are also possible.

Q: Can you develop immunity to Campylobacter infections?
A: Immunity is acquired after one or more infections.

Celiac Disease

 Basics

DESCRIPTION

Celiac disease is characterized by a permanent intolerance to gluten, leading to reversible changes of the small intestine. Gluten is a complex molecule found in wheat, rye, oats, and barley.

SIGNS AND SYMPTOMS

- Diarrhea
- Failure to thrive
- Vomiting
- Loss of appetite
- Delayed onset of puberty
- Dyspepsia, difficulty swallowing
- Arthritis and joint pain
- Mental retardation, neurologic problems

CAUSES

Various environmental factors that have been implicated include feeding practices, such as breast-feeding, and delay in exposure to gluten. Celiac disease may have a genetic component.

SCOPE

- 1 in 300 in the west of Ireland
- 1 in 6500 in Sweden
- Individuals of Asian or African descent are rarely afflicted.

 Diagnosis

QUESTIONS THE DOCTOR MAY ASK

N/A

WHAT THE DOCTOR LOOKS FOR

- Diversity in the presentation of celiac disease includes isolated short stature to the more classic description of "a grumpy, rickety, anemic, growth-retarded toddler with diarrhea, a potbelly, and muscle wasting."
- The most common age at which parents bring the child to a physician for these signs and symptoms is 1–5 years.

TESTS AND PROCEDURES

- Stool analysis
- Blood tests
- Small-bowel biopsy
- No specific test or combination of tests has been shown to be sufficient for diagnosis.

Treatment

GENERAL MEASURES

- Once diagnosis is confirmed, patients are given a strict gluten-free diet, with exclusion of all products containing oats, rye, wheat, and barley.
- Often, rice and corn may be used as alternative foods.
- The patient should be reassessed clinically and with repeat small-bowel biopsy.

ACTIVITY

N/A

DIET

Gluten-free diet

 ## Follow-Up

WHAT TO EXPECT

- Resolution of signs may take up to 2 years on a gluten-free diet.
- Patients who do not appear to respond may have poor compliance, complications of celiac disease, or another disease (e.g., inflammatory bowel disease).
- In addition to minimizing the symptoms and the complications of malabsorption, strict compliance with a gluten-free diet has been shown to decrease the risk of complications associated with celiac disease.

SIGNS TO WATCH

- Recurrence of diarrhea
- Appropraite weight gain

PREVENTION

N/A

 ## Common Questions and Answers

Q: What foods should be avoided in a gluten-free diet?
A: Products containing oats, rye, wheat, and barley. Often, rice and corn may be used as alternative foods.

Cellulitis

Basics

DESCRIPTION

Cellulitis is the inflammation and/or infection of the skin and subcutaneous tissues.

- Often classified by body area involved
- Most commonly occurs as a result of local trauma (abrasions, lacerations, bites, etc.)
- Periorbital cellulitis involves the eyelid and surrounding tissue, but not the eye itself.
- Local and distant spread of infection is possible.
- Extremity cellulitis may extend into the deep tissues to produce an arthritis.
- Cellulitis affecting the eye may be complicated by visual loss.

SIGNS AND SYMPTOMS

- An expanding, red, painful area of swelling
- Reddening, swelling, tenderness, and warmth
- Mild constitutional symptoms
- Serious systemic symptoms
- Redness and swelling of eyelid (periorbital cellulitis)

CAUSES

Bacterial infection

SCOPE

- Cellulitis that results from local skin trauma is by far the most common cause of cellulitis in children.
- Incidence of cellulitis that spreads throughout the body is decreasing.
- Periorbital cellulitis is common in children.

Diagnosis

QUESTIONS THE DOCTOR MAY ASK

- How fast is the redness spreading?
- Trauma history?
- Medications?
- Loss of function?

WHAT THE DOCTOR LOOKS FOR

- Signs and symptoms of cellulitis
- History of local trauma to the skin

TESTS AND PROCEDURES

- Culture of open wound
- Blood tests, blood culture
- Spinal tap
- X-rays
- Computed tomography (CT) of the head
- Sample of bone marrow

Treatment

GENERAL MEASURES

- Antibiotic drugs
- Abscesses should be surgically drained.

ACTIVITY

N/A

DIET

N/A

 ## Medications

COMMONLY PRESCRIBED DRUGS

Antibiotics

 ## Follow-Up

WHAT TO EXPECT

- Rapid, steady improvement should be expected.
- The prognosis for complete recovery is good as long as appropriate antimicrobials are administered in a timely fashion.

SIGNS TO WATCH

If daily improvement is not noted, inappropriate antimicrobial therapy, a deeper infection or abscess, or some other complication should be suspected.

PREVENTION

- Good wound care can prevent most cases of cellulitis.
- Cleanse all wounds thoroughly with soap and water, then cover with a clean, dry cloth.
- Topical antibiotic ointment is optional.

 ## Common Questions and Answers

Q: Is ophthalmology consultation necessary in all cases of periobital cellulitis?
A: Ophthalmology consultation is not necessaary in simple, uncomplicated cases of periorbital cellulitis that clearly have no associated proptosis, limitation in extraocular eye movement, or visual impairment that would suggest a more serious *orbital* cellulitis; if, however, the diagnosis is in question, consultation is indicated.

Cerebral Palsy

 Basics

DESCRIPTION

Cerebral palsy (CP) includes nonprogressive motor impairment syndromes that result from damage to or dysfunction of the developing brain.
- Subtypes are defined by type of neurologic impairment and anatomic distribution.
- CP subtypes may be associated with sensory disturbances, mental retardation, seizures, and other neurologic disorders.

SIGNS AND SYMPTOMS

- Sustained muscle contraction or spasms
- Spastic paralysis of half or the whole body
- Fluctuating muscle tone, rigidity
- Difficulty moving, walking

CAUSES

- Multiple causes
- In the majority of cases, the cause is not apparent.
- Prematurity
- Other abnormalities related to fetal development or birth

SCOPE

- The prevalence of cerebral palsy is approximately 2 in 1000 persons.
- Approximately 50% of cases are associated with prematurity.
- Increased incidence with multiple gestation (10% were twins in one study)
- More common among males

 Diagnosis

QUESTIONS THE DOCTOR MAY ASK

- Fetal development
- Premature delivery, neonatal resuscitation
- Postnatal: hospitalization for severe infection or trauma, failure to thrive
- Development: severe delay in motor milestones
- Family and social history

WHAT THE DOCTOR LOOKS FOR

- Physical examination
  - Drooling; increased muscle tone; increased reflexes; unequal muscle power for walking
  - Neurologic examination

TESTS AND PROCEDURES

- Hearing and vision tests
- Brain imaging
- Genetic and metabolic testing
- X-rays
- Blood tests
- Urodynamic studies
- Sleep study (polysomnography)
- Pulmonary function testing
- Electroencephalogram (EEG)

 Treatment

GENERAL MEASURES

- Family-centered care is directed toward optimizing function/minimizing handicap (habilitation).
- Interdisciplinary clinics provide multiple services (medical, surgical, therapy) coordinated with primary care physician.
- Primary care physician coordinates the goals of habilitation, therapy for seizure disorder, respiratory complications, and gastrointestinal issues.

Cerebral Palsy

- Education services should be tailored to the individual child. Despite recent emphasis on inclusion/mainstreaming, for many children, special education services are still required and appropriate.
- Physical, occupational, speech/language therapy, and other allied health professionals may provide therapy in home, school, and hospital settings. This therapy is directed primarily at improved functioning in the areas of mobility, self-care, and communication.
- Social services aid in the coordination of care.
- Medical subspecialists should be used according to needs of the individual child. These professionals may include developmental pediatricians, child neurologists, orthopedists, neurosurgeons, gastroenterologists, pulmonary medicine specialists, urologists, ophthalmologists, and otolaryngologists.

ACTIVITY

See General measures

DIET

N/A

 Medications

COMMONLY PRESCRIBED DRUGS

N/A

 Follow-Up

WHAT TO EXPECT

- Requirements for follow-up vary greatly with the degree of disability and the scope of impairments. An interdisciplinary clinic setting may be more appropriate for a child with severe CP.
- All children with CP should undergo audiologic and ophthalmologic assessment at the time of initial diagnosis.
- Early referral to a pediatric orthopedist is indicated, especially for monitoring of early hip problems.
- Early referral for developmental assessment is indicated to establish need for early intervention, to optimize development, and to promote family coping.

 Common Questions and Answers

Q: Do children with CP also have mental retardation?
A: Not necessarily. Although 50% have mental retardation, it is not a part of the definition of CP.

Q: What about surgery for CP?
A: Spasticity in the lower extremities may be addressed directly with selective surgery. Otherwise, surgical therapy is directed at associated conditions; many children with CP undergo orthopedic procedures for hip dislocation, release of contractures, and scoliosis. Surgery for correction of strabismus or placement of a gastrostomy tube is common.

Chickenpox

Basics

DESCRIPTION

Chickenpox, also called varicella, is a common, highly contagious disease of childhood marked by the development of crops of blisters on the skin and mucous membranes. It is caused by varicella zoster virus.

- The virus is spread directly by air or contact with blisters, or indirectly through freshly soiled articles.
- Outbreaks of chickenpox tend to occur from January to May.
- Incubation period is 14–16 days (range of 11 to 21 days).
- Patients are infectious from 24 hours before onset of the rash until the final lesions have crusted.
- Most people acquire chickenpox during childhood and develop lifelong immunity.
- Can be prevented by vaccine

SIGNS AND SYMPTOMS

- Prodromal symptoms: fever, malaise, lack of appetite, mild headache
- Characteristic rash: crops of "teardrop" blisters on reddened bases
- Blisters erupt in successive crops
- Develops from pimple to blister, then begins to crust
- The rash is present in various stages of development.
- Itching
- Rash usually begins on trunk, then spreads to face and scalp.
- Rash does not usually affect the arms or legs.
- Blisters are present on mucous membranes, such as the mouth and vagina.

CAUSES

Infection by the varicella zoster virus

SCOPE

- Chickenpox is common in the United States.
- Person-to-person transmission occurs by direct contact with varicella in an infected person's respiratory secretions.
- Varicella is most common during late winter and early spring.
- The introduction of one case of varicella into a home results in transmission of the virus to 98% of susceptible persons.
- Most reported cases occur between the ages of 5 and 9 years.
- Immunity from natural disease is usually life-long, but symptomatic reinfections do occur.
- Disease is also more severe in infants (less than 3 months old), adolescents, adults, those on steroids or long-term aspirin therapy, or those with pulmonary disorders.

Diagnosis

QUESTIONS THE DOCTOR MAY ASK

- Exposure
- Treatment of itching
- Prolonged headache
- Steroid medication
- Vaccination history
- Exposure to immunologic deficient patients

WHAT THE DOCTOR LOOKS FOR

Time of year, typical rash that has multiple stages identified, and history of not previously having had varicella usually make the diagnosis.

TESTS AND PROCEDURES

- None usually
- Analysis of blister fluid
- Blood tests

Treatment

GENERAL MEASURES

- Relief of symptoms
- Oatmeal bath for itching
- Topical anti-itch medication

ACTIVITY

Isolation of hospitalized patients

DIET

N/A

 ## Medications

COMMONLY PRESCRIBED DRUGS

- Acyclovir, vidarabine, famciclovir, foscarnet, and a number of antiviral agents have been shown in clinical trials to be effective against varicella zoster virus.
- Acyclovir is the drug of choice.
- Antihistamine for itching

 ## Follow-Up

WHAT TO EXPECT

- For normal, healthy individuals, follow-up is not necessary.
- For most children, chickenpox is a benign disease that lasts 6–8 days.
- 50–100 previously healthy children die each year from varicella, mostly caused by complications.
- With the advent of universal immunization, complications of varicella will decrease.

SIGNS TO WATCH

Scratching of lesions may result in infection.

PREVENTION

Varicella vaccine (Varivax)

 ## Common Questions and Answers

Q: When can the child return to school?
A: After the last lesion dries up to scab.

Q: How long will skin be discolored?
A: It may take months to return to usual skin color.

Child Abuse

 Basics

DESCRIPTION

- Child abuse is intentional injury of children at the hands of their caretakers.
- Physical abuse is legally defined by state laws.
- May result in death, mental retardation, cerebral palsy, seizures, learning disabilities, and emotional problems
- Child abuse is associated with domestic violence, sexual abuse, neglect, emotional abuse, juvenile delinquency, poverty, and parental substance abuse, including alcohol.

SIGNS AND SYMPTOMS

- Bruises, particularly in different stages of healing
- Burns, such as immersion burn
- Retinal bleeding
- Oral injuries
- Palpable rib fractures
- Abdominal injuries
- Genital injuries
- Broken bones
- Growth failure

CAUSES

- Multiple factors
- Include social, family, and individual factors
- Associated with poverty, family stress, family isolation

SCOPE

- Approximately 250,000 substantiated cases identified in the United States each year
- Almost 2000 deaths each year, by conservative estimates
- Parents who were abused as children are at much greater risk for abusing their own children. It is estimated that 30% of abused children become abusive parents.

 Diagnosis

QUESTIONS THE DOCTOR MAY ASK

- How did the injury occur?
- Who saw injury?
- Any previous injuries?
- Evidence of bleeding disorder?
- Family history of bone disease?
- Special questions
  - ▶ Does the history provided fit the clinical picture?
  - ▶ Are the findings explained by any medical condition?

WHAT THE DOCTOR LOOKS FOR

- History provided does not correlate with findings.
- Denial of trauma to child
- Child's development not compatible with mechanism of injury described
- History of events changes with time.
- Unexpected delay in seeking care
- Indications of family stress, isolation, substance abuse, and violence

TESTS AND PROCEDURES

- Blood tests
- X-rays of bones and chest
- Urinalysis
- Spinal tap
- Toxicology screens
- Radionuclide bone scan
- Computed tomography (CT) and magnetic resonance imaging (MRI)

Treatment

GENERAL MEASURES

- Ensure life and safety of child.
- Provide first aid as needed.
- Parental consent is often not needed for child abuse evaluation.
- Report suspected abuse to local child welfare agency.
- Report abuse to law enforcement.
- Consult social worker.
- Children with head injury should be examined by an ophthalmologist.

ACTIVITY

N/A

DIET

N/A

Medications

COMMONLY PRESCRIBED DRUGS

- Dependent on injury sustained
- Pain medication

Follow-Up

WHAT TO EXPECT

- Cases are investigated by child welfare agents and/or the police.
- Need for foster care placement, ongoing supervision decided by investigators
- Changes in family functioning often require intensive, long-term intervention.
- Improvement of individual injuries varies according to the injury; family functioning may improve with intervention for some families, but may never improve for others.

SIGNS TO WATCH

Noncompliance with medical follow-up or further injuries to child may indicate ongoing abuse, parental substance abuse, etc.

PREVENTION

Much of what is considered prevention is actually early intervention in high-risk families. Primary prevention would include universal parenting education and home visitation for all families. Currently, families thought to be at risk for abuse are identified and offered services.

Common Questions and Answers

Q: Does retinal bleeding indicate physical abuse?
A: Not necessarily. Retinal bleeding may be seen in a variety of diseases and in some normal newborns. Retinal bleeding occurs in approximately 30% of newborns delivered vaginally. In these children, the condition usually resolves in a few days, but it may rarely last for 5 to 6 weeks. Outside of the newborn period, severe accidental and inflicted injury is the leading cause of retinal bleeding in children. Retinal bleeding may also result from increased intracranial pressure, severe hypertension, carbon monoxide poisoning, blood-clotting disorders, and other conditions.

Q: When is a child abuse report filed?
A: Whenever there is a *suspicion*, based on the history, physical examination, laboratory data, and/or psychosocial assessment, that a child's injuries or illnesses were a result of abuse or neglect. Certainty regarding the diagnosis is not needed.

Q: Can the doctor be held liable for reports that are made but are not substantiated?
A: No. Physicians who report suspected abuse "in good faith" are protected from civil and criminal litigation arising from allegations of false reports.

Chlamydial Pneumonia

 Basics

DESCRIPTION

Chlamydial pneumonia is the most frequent cause of pneumonia without fever in infants. The chlamydia bacterium can infect the respiratory, genitourinary, and gastrointestinal systems and the eyes.

SIGNS AND SYMPTOMS

- Illness without fever
- Runny nose
- Cough
- Conjunctivitis (pink eye)
- Mild to severe respiratory distress
- Sore throat
- Hoarseness
- Cough
- Fever

CAUSE

Chlamydial infection, acquired from an infected mother during vaginal birth

SCOPE

- *Chlamydia trachomatis* is the most common sexually transmitted disease in the United States.
- Chlamydial infection in infants usually develops under 2 months of age (can range from 3 weeks to 6 months old).
- Reported as the most common cause of pneumonia in infants under 6 months of age (accounts for 25 to 45% of cases).
- 50% of neonates born to infected mothers via vaginal delivery acquire Chlamydia.

 Diagnosis

QUESTIONS THE DOCTOR MAY ASK

- Were cultures of vagina obtained at birth?
- Onset of symptoms?
- Presence of pink eye?
- Respiratory problem?
- Cough?

WHAT THE DOCTOR LOOKS FOR

Signs and symptoms of chlamydial infection or pneumonia
- Fever
- Cough
- Labored breathing

TESTS AND PROCEDURES

- Isolation of organism in culture
- Blood tests
- Chest X-ray
- Measurement of oxygen by finger probe

 Treatment

GENERAL MEASURES

- Fluids
- General nutrition

ACTIVITY

N/A

DIET

N/A

Medications

COMMONLY PRESCRIBED DRUGS

Antibiotics

 Follow-Up

WHAT TO EXPECT

- Recovery is usually slow.
- Cough and malaise may persist for several weeks.
- The outcome, in general, is good.
- Infection has been associated with an increased risk of developing asthma.

 Common Questions and Answers

Q: When a patient is infected with *Chlamydia trachomatis,* should any contacts be treated?
A: The mother and her sexual partner need to be treated.

Q: Is isolation of the patient required?
A: Isolation is not needed for pneumonia. Body fluid precautions are required for patients with conjunctivitis.

Chronic Active Hepatitis

 Basics

DESCRIPTION

Chronic active hepatitis (CAH) is a continuous inflammation of the liver leading to cirrhosis, liver failure, and death, and is often associated with autoimmune disease.

SIGNS AND SYMPTOMS

- Loss of appetite
- Malaise
- Nausea
- Vomiting
- Jaundice

CAUSES

- Autoimmune disorder
- Consequence of viral infection

SCOPE

Type II is autoimmune hepatitis. It occurs in 5 of 1,000,000 people, with an 8:1 ratio of female to male patients.

 Diagnosis

QUESTIONS THE DOCTOR MAY ASK

- Anorexia?
- Nausea?
- Vomiting?
- Jaundice?

WHAT THE DOCTOR LOOKS FOR

- Clinical features are often indistinguishable from acute viral hepatitis.
- Other patients have a more insidious course, without prominent signs and symptoms.
- Jaundice and enlarged liver and spleen
- Frequent findings of chronic liver disease
- Arthritis
- Inflammatory bowel disease

TESTS AND PROCEDURES

- Blood tests to test liver function, hepatitis titers, immune status
- Liver biopsy
- Ultrasound

Treatment

GENERAL MEASURES

- Therapy is continued until there is a clinical remission of symptoms.
- Liver biopsy is often repeated before therapy is tapered off.
- Surgery or liver transplantation may be required.

ACTIVITY

N/A

DIET

Good nutrition

 ## Medications

COMMONLY PRESCRIBED DRUGS

- Prednisone or prednisolone
- Azathioprine
- Cyclosporine and intravenous immunoglobulins have been used.

 ## Follow-Up

WHAT TO EXPECT

- Some children may develop acute liver failure.
- Children with autoimmune hepatitis have a wide spectrum of onset, from severe, progressive liver disease to symptomless liver enlargement to clinical and biochemical clues suggestive of acute viral hepatitis.
- Cirrhosis may develop aggressively.

SIGNS TO WATCH

- Increased lethargy
- Jaundice
- Loss of appetite
- Abdominal size
- Bleeding

PREVENTION

N/A

 ## Common Questions and Answers

Q: Do children need to be treated with steroids and other drugs?
A: Yes, children who present with signs and symptoms of chronic autoimmune hepatitis are treated as aggressively as adults. Steroids and other immunosuppressive drugs are used as in adults.

Cleft Lip

 Basics

DESCRIPTION

A cleft lip (CL) is a deformity of the upper lip that may include a defect of skin, muscle, mucous surfaces, the gums, and bone. The cleft may be on one side of the face or both sides. A cleft palate (CP) is usually a visible separation between the two halves of the roof of the mouth, involving mucous surfaces, muscle, and often the bones of the hard palate.

- May be complicated by airway obstruction or feeding disorders
- Approximately one-third of patients with cleft palate have other defects, such as central nervous system, heart, and urinary tract malformations, and club foot.

SIGNS AND SYMPTOMS

Interruption of the normal contour and surface of the lip or roof of the mouth

CAUSES

- Abnormal embryonic development
- One-third of patients with cleft lip and/or palate have a positive family history.
- Two-thirds of cases have no clear genetic basis and are presumed to be environmental. Clefts may be attributable to alcohol, anticonvulsants (phenytoin), and isotretinoin. Isolated clefting has not been associated with prenatal exposure to a single substance.

SCOPE

Incidence of cleft lip with or without cleft palate is 1 in 700 births.

 Diagnosis

QUESTIONS THE DOCTOR MAY ASK

- Stress in pregnancy
- Family problems
- Heart problems
- Experience with other patients with CP or CL

WHAT THE DOCTOR LOOKS FOR

- Incomplete or complete cleft of lip, hard or soft palate, or uvula
- Associated anomalies of the face, heart, and extremities that may indicate a cleft syndrome
- Prenatal exposure to alcohol, cigarettes, phenytoin, isotretinoin; family history of cleft lip or cleft palate; speech problems in first-degree relative
- Ear disease
- Nutrition
- Growth pattern
- Speech development

TESTS AND PROCEDURES

- Complete ophthalmologic exam
- Hearing tests
- Blood tests
- Genetic screening
- Echocardiography, kidney ultrasound, intravenous pyelogram, if indicated

 Treatment

GENERAL MEASURES

- Airway management, prone positioning if tongue is causing airway obstruction
- Patients with cleft lip may have significant feeding problems because of inability to suck.
- Surgery: Palate repair is generally done before 1 year of age to decrease speech and language difficulties.
- Orthodontics may include devices to help feeding and speech.

- Multiple ear infections may require prolonged use of tubes to prevent hearing impairment.
- Delays in speech and language development may require detailed evaluation, early intervention programs, and speech therapy.
- Poor dentition, bite problems, gingivitis, and crowding have been noted.
- Behavior disorders and psychosocial adjustment disorders may require attention.
- Multidisciplinary team approach, including a pediatrician, plastic surgeon, speech pathologist, orthodontist, pediatric dentist, psychologist, social worker, nurse practitioner, anthropologist (facial growth specialist), geneticist, support group

ACTIVITY

N/A

DIET

N/A

 ## Medications

COMMONLY PRESCRIBED DRUGS

N/A

 ## Follow-Up

WHAT TO EXPECT

- Prognosis is good for normal growth and development with long-term follow-up by a multidisciplinary team and with good parental support.
- 30% of patients may require additional surgery after initial repair.
- Otitis media (middle ear infection) is more common with cleft palate.

 ## Common Questions and Answers

Q: Will my child look normal?
A: All cleft lip repairs will leave some type of permanent scar, with potential asymmetry that may benefit from later additional lip scar revision. The goal is to create a lip that does not attract undue attention. The nose is often the most difficult to correct.

Q: Will my child speak normally?
A: Most children will achieve normal speech, but may require additional speech therapy to achieve this goal.

Clubfoot

 Basics

DESCRIPTION

Clubfoot is a congenital or neuromuscular deformity of the foot and ankle.

SIGNS AND SYMPTOMS

- Deformity of the foot—toe is pointed down and cannot be moved to normal position; sole of foot faces midline
- Abnormal bone formation
- Loss of function

CAUSES

Most cases are of unknown cause.

SCOPE

- Prevalence of clubfoot is 1–1.4 per 1000 live births.
- The risk of deformity increases by 20 to 30 times when there is an affected first-degree relative.
- More common among males

 Diagnosis

QUESTIONS THE DOCTOR MAY ASK

- Fetal movement
- Family history

WHAT THE DOCTOR LOOKS FOR

- Family history
- Onset of deformity

TESTS AND PROCEDURES

X-rays

 Treatment

GENERAL MEASURES

- Initial treatment is manipulation and casting.
- Failure to correct the deformity completely by manipulation within 3 to 9 months should lead to surgical treatment.

ACTIVITY

N/A

DIET

N/A

Medications

COMMONLY PRESCRIBED DRUGS
N/A

 Follow-Up

WHAT TO EXPECT
- Most surgeons cast the feet for 3 months after surgery; some brace the feet for 6 months.
- Depending on the severity of the deformity and treatment, a difference between the feet of one to two shoe sizes and even a leg-length discrepancy are present.

SIGNS TO WATCH
N/A

PREVENTION
N/A

 Common Questions and Answers

Q: What percentage of clubfeet are treated successfully by casting?
A: To some extent, the amount of success depends on how much correction is desired. Positional clubfeet are likely to improve with casting in perhaps 80% of cases. Rigid clubfeet are much less likely to be corrected by casting. The success rate in the rigid feet is likely to be approximately 10–20%.

Q: What will be the permanent disability of a congenital clubfoot deformity?
A: Although casting and surgical correction of a congenital clubfoot can realign the bones, the surgery does little to correct the underlying neuromuscular problems. As a result, all children with rigid clubfeet are likely to have a leg-length inequality (usually less than 1.5 inches), a smaller foot (usually one to two sizes), calf narrowing that cannot be improved significantly with exercise, and joint stiffness. Even children with optimal realignment of the deformity note inability to perform gymnastic activities or running activities requiring normal range of motion of the ankle and foot. Many of these children report an inability to keep up with their peer group during adolescent and young adult sports activities.

Q: How soon should an infant with congenital clubfoot be referred to an orthopedic surgeon?
A: If casting is to be even partially successful, cast treatment should begin within the first week or two of life. Clearly, medical and life-threatening conditions take precedence over the treatment of the clubfoot. Casting should begin as soon as is practical. It may even be possible to begin taping of the foot as an alternative to casting. Referral to an orthopedic surgeon should therefore be as soon as is practical.

Colic

Basics

DESCRIPTION

Colic is a poorly defined and incompletely understood state of excessive crying in young infants who are otherwise well. There is no standard definition of colic. The quality of crying of colicky infants is not different from that of noncolicky infants, but the quantity of crying is considerably more than the average.

SIGNS AND SYMPTOMS

More than 3 hours a day of irritability, fussing, or crying on more than 3 days in any 1 week during the first 3–4 months of life in an infant who is otherwise healthy and well-fed. The baby usually turns red and draws legs upward.

CAUSES

- No single cause always found
- Typically, problem lies in interaction between factors in infant and environment

SCOPE

- Typically begins shortly after baby comes home from hospital
- Can last until 3 to 4 months of age if not managed successfully
- If excessive crying lasts after 4 months, other diagnoses should be considered.

Diagnosis

QUESTIONS THE DOCTOR MAY ASK

- How do the parents react to crying?
- What have they done to stop the crying?
- What do they know about colic?
- How is the family handling the crying?
- What are the parents' support systems?
- Intensity, duration, and frequency of crying?
- Description and demonstration of soothing techniques?
- Information on the baby's temperament?
- Medical history?

WHAT THE DOCTOR LOOKS FOR

- Physical examination—looks for red eye (glaucona)

TESTS AND PROCEDURES

- No tests are indicated unless specifically suggested by history and physical examination.
- Attempts at management over the telephone without a physical examination are not likely to be successful.

Treatment

GENERAL MEASURES

- The most effective form of treatment is counseling, which should consist of these main points:
  - ▶ *The infant is not sick.* Although crying may be persistent, the infant has no evidence of a physical problem. Therefore, there is no proof the infant is having pain, just distress. The infant is probably just over-aroused and tired.
  - ▶ *Education about infant crying.* Parents need to know how much normal infants cry and how they vary in sensitivity, irritability, and soothability. The way parents react to their infants can affect amount of crying. Parents often do not understand that a common reason for infant crying is fatigue and a need to be left alone.
  - ▶ *The excessive crying can be reduced.* Parents have to learn to tune in more sensitively to the infants' needs and to be more effectively responsive to them.
- Basic strategy
  - ▶ Soothing by a pacifier, repetitive sound, or a hot-water bottle
  - ▶ Stimulate less by decreasing the picking up, holding, and feeding the infant when it is not appropriate
  - ▶ A quiet environment, correction of any faulty feeding techniques, and a minimum of unnecessary handling without changing the composition of the feedings
- Expression of optimism by pediatrician about the immediate outcome is justified and in itself improves chances of success. Simply saying that it will be gone by 3 to 4 months of age is not comforting.
- Extra carrying does not help.
- Formula changes are frequently attempted by physicians hoping for a simple solution, but they rarely are effective. Sometimes they seem to be helpful for a few days, only to cease being so a day or two later.
- Almost any procedure done with conviction is likely to be followed by a temporary reduction in crying because of the placebo effect.

ACTIVITY

No need to change formula, but this is frequently done

DIET

N/A

Follow-Up

WHAT TO EXPECT

- It is important for parents of an excessively fussy baby to keep in close touch with their pediatrician. Telephone contact every 2–3 days is essential until improvement. Reexamination is rarely needed.
- Colic usually goes away by itself by 3 to 4 months of age, and little can be done to change that pattern. Several studies report that colic can be reduced within 2 to 3 days if management such as that described above is used. Some infants take longer, but virtually all respond to suitable management. The long-term outcome of these infants has not been adequately studied.

SIGNS TO WATCH

N/A

PREVENTION

N/A

Common Questions and Answers

Q: What is wrong with my baby? What can we do to relieve the pain? Why is he/she so gassy? Shouldn't we strengthen the formula? You mean it's all my fault? Will this ever stop? What will he/she be like later?
A: All the answers are to be found above.

Congenital Gonococcal Infection

 Basics

DESCRIPTION

Gonorrhea, a disease caused by the bacteria *Neisseria gonorrhoeae,* can be acquired by an infant from an infected mother. This type of infection is called congenital gonococcal infection. Neonatal gonococcal diseases include eye infection, scalp abscess (complication after fetal scalp monitoring), and, rarely, vaginitis or systemic disease.

SIGNS AND SYMPTOMS

- Infants:
  - ▶ Eye infection
  - ▶ Pneumonia
  - ▶ Vaginal discharge
  - ▶ Rectal infection
  - ▶ Throat infection
  - ▶ Other forms of infection

SCOPE

N/A

 Diagnosis

QUESTIONS THE DOCTOR MAY ASK

N/A

WHAT THE DOCTOR LOOKS FOR

- Signs and symptoms of gonococcal disease

TESTS AND PROCEDURES

- Blood tests
- Culture of infectious fluids

Treatment

GENERAL MEASURES

- Antibiotic therapy
- Neonates with eye infection should have their eyes frequently irrigated with sterile saline until drainage has ceased.
- Contact isolation precautions for all patients with gonococcal disease in the neonatal age group

ACTIVITY

N/A

DIET

N/A

 ## Medications

COMMONLY PRESCRIBED DRUGS

Antibiotics (e.g., ceftriaxone, cefotaxime)

 ## Follow-Up

WHAT TO EXPECT

A good outcome depends on diagnosis and effective eradication of infection prior to the development of complications.

SIGNS TO WATCH

N/A

PREVENTION

N/A

 ## Common Questions and Answers

N/A

Congenital Hip Dysplasia

 Basics

DESCRIPTION

Congenital hip dysplasia comprises a range of congenital hip disorders, including dislocation of the hip. If left untreated, congenital hip dysplasia results in limp, pain, and accelerated degenerative disease of the hip.

SIGNS AND SYMPTOMS

- Excessive flexibility of hip
- Legs of different length
- Foot pointed in or out

CAUSES

- Breech birth
- Lax ligaments
- Connective tissue disorder
- Other factors

SCOPE

- The incidence of hip dysplasia is 0.5–2% of live births.
- True dislocation of hip occurs in 0.1–0.2% of live births.

 Diagnosis

QUESTIONS THE DOCTOR MAY ASK

N/A

WHAT THE DOCTOR LOOKS FOR

- Breech birth
- Family history of hip dysplasia (10–20% of patients have family history)
- Physical examination: symmetry of legs and skin, hip joint tests, inequality of skinfolds in leg

TESTS AND PROCEDURES

- X-rays
- Ultrasound

Treatment

GENERAL MEASURES

- Triple diaper is not effective in moderate or severe dysplasia.
- Pavlik harness is effective if used before 6 months of age.
- Closed or open reduction is necessary if diagnosis/therapy has been delayed beyond 6 months.

ACTIVITY

N/A

DIET

N/A

 ## Follow-Up

WHAT TO EXPECT

- In children treated early (age less than 4 months), duration of splinting is 3–4 weeks.
- If diagnosed early, prognosis is uniformly excellent.

SIGNS TO WATCH

- Unequal growth of leg
- Decreased range of motion of leg

PREVENTION

N/A

 ## Common Questions and Answers

Q: Is this a vitamin deficiency?
A: No.

Q: Did something that happened during pregnancy cause this?
A: Is there something that happened to make you ask this? (Not known cause of most cases.) Some have lax ligaments.

Q: Is this the same as "hip click"?
A: Hip click is a clicking sound when knees are moved outward. The lax ligaments allow head of leg to move out of hip joint. These usually improve.

Congenital Hypothyroidism

 ## Basics

DESCRIPTION

Congenital hypothyroidism is absence or malfunction of the thyroid gland. If untreated, it can lead to severe mental retardation (cretinism), poor motor development, and poor growth.

SIGNS AND SYMPTOMS

- Weakness, lethargy
- Prolonged jaundice
- Poor feeding
- Constipation
- Low body temperature
- Hoarse cry
- Distended abdomen
- Umbilical hernia
- Coarse facial features
- Large tongue

CAUSES

Absence or other disorder of the thyroid gland

SCOPE

- In North America, the incidence is 1 per 3700 live births.
- More common in females

 ## Diagnosis

QUESTIONS THE DOCTOR MAY ASK

- Constipation
- Prolonged jaundice in newborn
- Family history of thyroid disease
- Activity level
- Developmental assessment
  - Most children are diagnosed by the neonatal screening.
  - Maternal medications
  - Birth history
  - Thyroid disorders among family members

WHAT THE DOCTOR LOOKS FOR

- Signs and symptoms of congenital hypothyroidism

TESTS AND PROCEDURES

- Blood tests of thyroid function
- Thyroid scan

 ## Treatment

GENERAL MEASURES

- Drug therapy
- Treatment may be lifelong.

ACTIVITY

N/A

DIET

No restrictions

Medications

COMMONLY PRESCRIBED DRUGS

L-thyroxine

 ## Follow-Up

WHAT TO EXPECT

- Most children have no symptoms at time of diagnosis.
- Parents may note an increase in activity, improvement in feeding, and increased urination and bowel movements soon after starting treatment.
- Prognosis is excellent if treatment is started within first 4 weeks of life.

SIGNS TO WATCH

Poor growth

PREVENTION

N/A

 ## Common Questions and Answers

Q: Will my child be retarded?
A: It depends on when the diagnosis was made and how quickly treatment was started. Some long-term studies have suggested an increase in learning disabilities when compared to siblings even in patients treated within the first 4 weeks of life.

Q: What if I forget a dose?
A: Give as soon as you remember. If it is the next day, give two doses.

Q: Are there side effects from the medication?
A: No. The tablet contains only the hormone that your child's thyroid is not making.

Constipation

Basics

DESCRIPTION

Constipation is a combination of changes in the frequency, size, consistency, and ease of stool passage, which leads to an overall decrease in volume of bowel movements. "Normal" toilet habits vary over a wide range; occasional episodes of constipation are to be expected.

SIGNS AND SYMPTOMS

- Less frequency of defecation than usual
- Harder stool than usual
- Smaller stool than usual
- Impaction of stool
- Lack of consistent urgency to stool
- Difficulty expelling feces
- Painful evacuation of feces
- Sensation of incomplete emptying of the bowel
- Abdominal fullness
- Painful spasm of the rectum

CAUSES

- Fiber poor diet
- Inadequate fluid intake
- Electrolyte disturbance
- Hormonal disturbance (hypothyroidism, diabetes)
- Congenital conditions of rectum and large intestine—rectal fissure; Hirschsprung disease
- Other illness, injury, or debility
- Other bowel conditions
- Side effect of drugs (e.g., anticholinergic agents, opiates)
- Chronic abuse of laxatives or cathartics
- Psychiatric, cultural, emotional, environmental factors

SCOPE

Constipation is common.

Diagnosis

QUESTIONS THE DOCTOR MAY ASK

Question: Frequent urination, bed wetting, or urinary tract infections?
Significance: Seen frequently with chronic constipation
Question: Soiling?
Significance: Soiling occurs if stool is impacted.
Question: Rectal sensation?
Significance: Patients with long-standing constipation or withholding who develop a dilated rectum often lose the sensation of rectal distention.
Question: History of painful BM or rectal fissure?
Significance: Could have been the beginning of withholding caused by fear of painful BM
Question: Personality of child?
Significance: Common age for onset of stool withholding is 2–4 years of age, i.e., at the time of toilet training. The child wants to control the parents and his or her environment. Some children are too busy playing to take the time to have a BM. Some children do not want to use the toilet in school because of hygiene issues.
Question: Stressful events, e.g., new sibling, death in family?
Significance: Can result in stool withholding and constipation
Question: Unsteady or clumsy toilet training?
Significance: May suggest neuromuscular problems. Some children with soiling have a history of difficult toilet training or failure of toilet training.
Question: Diet history or caloric intake, fluid, milk, caffeine, and fiber intake?
Significance: Excessive amounts of milk (calcium) and caffeine may be constipating in some individuals.

Constipation

WHAT THE DOCTOR LOOKS FOR

- Physical examination
- Rectal fissure
- Stone in rectum
- Innervation of rectal area
- Abdominal examination
- Mass of stone in left side

TESTS AND PROCEDURES

- Abdominal x-rays
- Barium enema
- Evaluation of rectal muscles
- Rectal biopsy

Treatment

GENERAL MEASURES

- Proper diet, bowel training, and use of bulk-forming supplements are important.
- Attempt to eliminate medications that may cause or worsen constipation.
- Increase fluid intake.
- Modify diet.
- Use enemas or suppositories if other remedies fail.

ACTIVITY

Exercise is encouraged.

DIET

- Increase fiber.
- Maintain adequate hydration.

Medications

COMMONLY PRESCRIBED DRUGS

- Stool softener
- Mineral oil

Follow-Up

WHAT TO EXPECT

Constipation that is occasional, brief, and responsive to simple measures is harmless. Habitual constipation can be a lifelong nuisance.

SIGNS TO WATCH

Fecal soiling

PREVENTION

Diet—well-balanced with fiber, vegetables. Substitute sugar-coated cereals with bran-like cereals.

Common Questions and Answers

Q: Why not give an enema every day or so?
A: This empties the bowel but does not require muscle tone and use of natural urges.

Q: Why do you suggest fluid and fiber?
A: These items will keep stool soft and will stretch the intestine to signal time for defecation. Without these products, the stool becomes hard and dry, making it difficult to defecate.

Croup

 Basics

DESCRIPTION

Croup is an acute viral infection of the respiratory system.

SIGNS AND SYMPTOMS

- Barking cough
- High-pitched sound upon breathing (stridor)
- Hoarseness
- Sore throat
- Fever
- Difficulty swallowing
- Respiratory distress: rapid breathing rate; bluish discoloration around lips, eyes, and nail beds (cyanosis)

CAUSES

Viral infection

SCOPE

- Peak age range: 6 months to 3 years of age
- 80% of cases occur in children less than 5 years of age.
- More common in males than females
- Fall and winter predominance

 Diagnosis

QUESTIONS THE DOCTOR MAY ASK

- Did onset of stridor occur while child was playing with toys or eating?
- Did symptoms improve with shower mist?
- Did stridor awaken a previously well child from sleep?

WHAT THE DOCTOR LOOKS FOR

- Onset and progression of symptoms
- Physical examination
- Assess quality of respiration
- Fatigue
- Cyanosis
- Agitation

TESTS AND PROCEDURES

X-rays of neck

 Treatment

GENERAL MEASURES

- Humidity: a steam-filled bathroom or humidifier
- Fluids

ACTIVITY

N/A

DIET

N/A

Medications

COMMONLY PRESCRIBED DRUGS

- Epinephrine
- Steroids
- Dexamethasone

 ## Follow-Up

WHAT TO EXPECT

- Patients with croup generally improve over 3 to 5 days.
- Most patients recover completely.
- Most patients do not require hospitalization or intubation.
- Studies have shown that some children with a history of croup have a higher likelihood of asthma.

SIGNS TO WATCH

Worsening respiratory distress, high fevers, and increased secretions, irritability, fatigue

 ## Common Questions and Answers

Q: Why do you ask about playing with toys?
A: Swallowing of small toys, which lodges in airway, may cause similar symptoms is croup?

Q: Why is irritability a bad sign?
A: It may indicate poor oxygenation, a sign of respiratory failure.

Q: Why does steam seem to make it better?
A: Not clear, but it works.

Q: When is the worst time of the day for a patient with croup?
A: Nighttime. It usually gets better at dawn.

Cryptorchidism

 Basics

DESCRIPTION

Cryptorchidism is a condition in which the testicles have not descended into the scrotum.

SIGNS AND SYMPTOMS

Undescended testicles

CAUSES

- Hormone disorder
- Anatomic abnormalities—poorly developed testes

SCOPE

- Incidence greater in premature infants: 3.4% in full-term infants; 17% in premature infants weighing 2 to 2.5 kilograms; 100% in infants weighing 900 grams
- 0.7% incidence in children more than 1 year old and adults

 Diagnosis

QUESTIONS THE DOCTOR MAY ASK

- Did you ever see or feel testicle with scrotum?
- Premature birth?

WHAT THE DOCTOR LOOKS FOR

- The absence of testicles in the scrotum
- Will differentiate undescended testicles from testes that retract into abdomen—from cold air or cold fingers of examiner.

TESTS AND PROCEDURES

- Blood tests
- Venography   } not done usually
- Laparoscopy

Treatment

GENERAL MEASURES

- Conservative therapy: hormones
- Observe to see if growth and weight increase will allow testes to drop into scrotum—will not occur after 1 year of age
- Hormones—human chronic gonadotrophinor leutenizing hormone—releasing hormone
- Surgery

ACTIVITY

N/A

DIET

N/A

 ## Follow-Up

WHAT TO EXPECT

- Treatment may preserve fertility.
- In patients in which both testicles are affected and treated, one-third are fertile.
- 20–44% increased risk of cancer in third and fourth decades of life in patients with undescended testes, especially if the condition untreated or corrected after or during puberty.
- Cancer is found in 2–3% of all men with a history of cryptorchidism.

SIGNS TO WATCH

N/A

PREVENTION

N/A

 ## Common Questions and Answers

Q: Why will not all testes eventually drop?
A: some are not formed normally, so they do not grow and descend.

Q: Why not fix the problem at birth?
A: Some will eventually drop into scrotum.

Cystic Fibrosis

 Basics

DESCRIPTION

Cystic fibrosis (CF) is a genetic disorder characterized by chronic obstructive lung disease, pancreatic deficiency, and elevated concentration of salts in the sweat.

SIGNS AND SYMPTOMS

- Sweat glands
  - Increased concentrations of salt
  - Dehydration with heat and infections
- Respiratory system
  - Wheezing
  - Chronic cough
  - Difficulty breathing
  - Rapid breathing
  - Barrel chest
  - Repeated bouts of bronchitis or pneumonia
- Gastrointestinal system
  - Failure to thrive
  - Chronic, recurrent abdominal pain
  - Gastroesophageal reflux
  - Voracious appetite before treatment
  - A sensation of fullness in the abdomen
  - Frequent, bulky, foul-smelling, pale stool
- Others
  - Delayed weight gain during growth and development
  - Retarded bone growth
  - Delayed sexual development
  - Infertility in males
  - Nasal polyps

CAUSES

Inherited genetic defect

SCOPE

- 1 per 2500 in Caucasian population
- 1 per 17,000 in African-American population
- Rarely seen in African blacks and Asians
- Most common severe inherited disease in the Caucasian population

 Diagnosis

QUESTIONS THE DOCTOR MAY ASK

- Family history?
- Problem with passing stool at birth?
- Is stool foul smelling?
- Frequent cough and respiratory infection?
- Growth patterns?

WHAT THE DOCTOR LOOKS FOR

Common signs and symptoms of cystic fibrosis
- Small size
- Protuberant abdomen
- Increased chest diameter
- Nasal polyps
- Enlarged salivary gland

TESTS AND PROCEDURES

- Sweat test
- Sputum cultures
- Pulmonary function tests
- Pancreatic function tests
- Chest X-ray

 Treatment

GENERAL MEASURES

- Supportive care
- Respiratory therapy
- Medications
- Usually lifelong nutritional support required
- Duration of antibiotic therapy is controversial; more chronic use is required as pulmonary function deteriorates.
- Specialized care should take place at a cystic fibrosis center.
- Frequency of visits depends on severity of illness; usually every 2–4 months.

ACTIVITY

Chest physiotherapy with postural drainage

DIET

- Pancreatic enzyme replacement therapy
- Vitamin supplements
- High-calorie diet with nutritional supplements

Medications

COMMONLY PRESCRIBED DRUGS

- Cephalexin
- Cefaclor
- Trimethoprim-sulfamethoxazole
- Chloramphenicol
- Ciprofloxacin
- Intravenous antibiotics
- Aerosolized bronchodilator therapy
- *N*-acetylcysteine (Mucomyst)
- rhDNase (Dornase)

 ## Follow-Up

WHAT TO EXPECT

- Long-term prognosis is poor.
- Current mean life span is 29 years.
- The mean age of survival has been increasing for the past three decades.

SIGNS TO WATCH

Growth, respiratory distress, diet, psychosocial development

PREVENTION

N/A

 ## Common Questions and Answers

Q: Should relatives be tested?
A: All siblings should have a sweat test. It is assumed that the parents are healthy carriers if they are asymptomatic.

Q: How well will a child do?
A: The course of the illness is variable. It is impossible to predict the course of the disease in a specific person.

Cytomegalovirus Infection

 Basics

DESCRIPTION

Cytomegalovirus (CMV) is a common virus that is a member of the herpes family. The virus often establishes latency in the body. Infection with CMV during pregnancy can be extremely hazardous to the fetus.

SIGNS AND SYMPTOMS

- May have no symptoms
- Fatigue
- Nausea
- Vomiting
- Bone pain
- Chills
- Fever
- Diarrhea
- Jaundice
- Difficulty breathing
- Pneumonia (fever, cough, chills, chest pain)
- Ulcers of gastrointestinal tract

CAUSES

Viral infection

SCOPE

- Prevalence varies with socioeconomic status.
- Less than 50% of middle and about 80% of lower socioeconomic status adults test positive for CMV.
- Increased rates of primary infection seen in early childhood, adolescence, and child-bearing years.
- Transmission may occur via contact with infected respiratory secretions, urine or breast milk, sexual contact, organ transplantation, or infusion of infected blood products.

 Diagnosis

QUESTIONS THE DOCTOR MAY ASK

History: day-care attendance; recent blood transfusion; use of immunosuppressive medications; prolonged fever; blurred vision; cough, difficult breathing, wheezing; vomiting, abdominal pain, diarrhea (watery or bloody)

WHAT THE DOCTOR LOOKS FOR

Physical examination for source of fever; chest examination; jaundice

TESTS AND PROCEDURES

- Viral culture
- Blood tests

 Treatment

GENERAL MEASURES

N/A

ACTIVITY

N/A

DIET

N/A

Medications

COMMONLY PRESCRIBED DRUGS

- Ganciclovir
- Foscarnet

 Follow-Up

WHAT TO EXPECT

Outcome depends on severity and type of infection.

SIGNS TO WATCH

N/A

PREVENTION

Body fluid precautions for hospitalized patients known to be shedding CMV

 Common Questions and Answers

Q: Should children with congenital CMV infection be excluded from day-care settings? **A:** No. Because of the high frequency of shedding of CMV in the urine and saliva of asymptomatic children, especially under 2 years of age, exclusion from out-of-home care is not justified for any child known to be infected with CMV. Careful attention to hygienic practices, especially hand washing, is important.

Dehydration

 ## Basics

DESCRIPTION

Dehydration is a negative balance of body fluid, usually expressed as a percentage of body weight. Mild, moderate, and severe dehydration correspond to deficits of 5%, 10%, and 15%, respectively.

SIGNS AND SYMPTOMS

- Lethargy, irritability, thirst
- Rapid heart rate, low blood pressure and/or increase in heart rate when standing, rapid breathing rate
- Mottling, tenting of skin when pinched
- Decreased or absent tears; sunken eyes
- Decreased urine output
- Dry or parched mucous surfaces
- Sunken "soft spot" (fontanelle)

CAUSES

- Dehydration is caused by either excessive fluid losses or inadequate intake. Some causes of dehydration include
  - ▶ Gastrointestinal: Vomiting and diarrhea are the most common causes of dehydration in children.
  - ▶ Urinary: diabetes, diuretics ("water pills")
  - ▶ Insensible losses: sweating, fever, rapid breathing, warm room temperature, large burns
  - ▶ Poor intake: sore throat, loss of appetite, oral trauma, altered mental status
- Infants and debilitated patients are at particular risk because of lack of ability to satisfy their thirst freely.

SCOPE

- Approximately 10% of children in the United States with acute gastroenteritis develop at least mild dehydration.
- Although dehydration accounts for 10% of all nonsurgical hospital admissions for children under 5 years of age, up to 90% of cases can be managed on an outpatient basis.

 ## Diagnosis

QUESTIONS THE DOCTOR MAY ASK

- Signs and symptoms of dehydration
- Frequency and duration of vomiting and/or diarrhea
- Amount and type of liquids taken
- Frequency and quantity of urination (may be difficult to estimate in infants with diarrhea)
- How many diapers were changed
- Dark yellow urine

WHAT THE DOCTOR LOOKS FOR

- Fever
- Exertion or heat exposure
- Rapid pulse rate
- Change in activity; increased sleepiness
- Dry skin
- Tears
- Moist or dry mouth
- Change in blood pressure when standing up compared to sitting down

TESTS AND PROCEDURES

- Blood tests
- Urinalysis

 ## Treatment

GENERAL MEASURES

- Oral rehydration therapy (ORT)
  - ▶ Most children can be managed successfully with ORT.
  - ▶ Use rehydration solution containing sugar and salt (Pedialyte, Ricelyte)
  - ▶ Begin with slow administration, with strict limits when vomiting is present (5 ml every 1–2 minutes). For infants, use a syringe or spoon rather than a bottle. After an hour, if the oral liquids have been tolerated, increase the volume and rate.

- ▶ Monitor weight, intake and output, and clinical signs. Failure of ORT includes intractable vomiting, clinical deterioration, or lack of improvement after 4 hours.
- Intravenous fluid therapy
- After rehydration, children with ongoing losses, as in gastroenteritis, should receive a maintenance solution in addition to regular feedings to maintain a positive fluid balance.
- Avoid clear liquids with excessive sugar, such as fruit juices, punches, and soft drinks, as these can promote even more fluid losses in the stool. In infants younger than 6 months old, do not give large amounts of plain water.

ACTIVITY

N/A

DIET

N/A

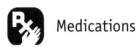 Medications

COMMONLY PRESCRIBED DRUGS

N/A

 Follow-Up

WHAT TO EXPECT

If dehydration is recognized early and treated promptly, most dehydrated children recover very well.

SIGNS TO WATCH

See Signs and symptoms

PREVENTION

- Maintain adequate fluid intake.
- Avoid prolonged exposure to high temperatures.
- Recognize the early signs of dehydration.

 Common Questions and Answers

Q: Can commercially available maintenance solutions be used for rehydration as well as maintenance?
A: Data suggest that commercial rehydration liquids are equally effective for rehydration as solutions with a higher sodium content.

Dermatitis

 Basics

DESCRIPTION

Dermatitis is an inflammatory reaction of the skin.

- Contact dermatitis is an inflammation in response to an external substance; the eruption may result from direct irritation of the skin or a delayed allergic reaction.
- Seborrheic dermatitis is a yellowish or reddish, scaly, greasy lesion located in areas of high concentrations of sebaceous glands (the scalp, face, behind the ear, and folds of skin). The term seborrhea refers to excessively oily skin.
- Atopic dermatitis or eczema is a chronic, itchy, bumpy eruption seen in persons with a personal or family history of asthma, allergies, hay fever, or rhinitis. There are often periodic flares of acute atopic dermatitis. It most commonly begins in infancy or early childhood.

SIGNS AND SYMPTOMS

- Atopic dermatitis
  - ▶ Itching
  - ▶ Reddened lesions that may ooze and crust
  - ▶ Scaling skin
  - ▶ Flushing of the face
  - ▶ Dry skin
- Contact dermatitis
  - ▶ Bumps, blisters, or rash surrounded by reddened skin
  - ▶ Crusting or oozing
  - ▶ Itching
  - ▶ Thickening of skin
  - ▶ Flaking, scaling
  - ▶ Fissuring
  - ▶ Areas of contact with offending agent (e.g., nail polish)
  - ▶ Linear lesions or welts
  - ▶ Lesions with sharp borders and sharp angles
- Seborrheic dermatitis
  - ▶ Cradle cap: greasy scaling of scalp
  - ▶ In adults: red, greasy, scaling patches of smooth skin; dandruff—like lesions

Dermatitis

CAUSES

- Contact dermatitis may be caused by poison ivy, leather dyes, oils from fruit peelings, harsh soaps, acids, certain foods, saliva, urine, and feces.
- Common allergens resulting in delayed hypersensitivity reactions include vinyl, metals (particularly nickel), antihistamines, and plastics in rubber products.
- Although it has been postulated that seborrheic dermatitis is initiated by a bacterial or fungal infection, this has not been proven and the specific cause is controversial.
- The cause of atopic dermatitis has multiple origins, with genetic, environmental, physiologic, and immunologic factors.

SCOPE

- Contact dermatitis can occur at any age, although young infant skin is more easily irritated by a primary irritant. Infants seem to be less likely to develop a delayed hypersensitivity response.
- Seborrheic dermatitis is first seen in infancy and usually spontaneously resolves by the end of the first year of life. It is not usually seen again until adolescence.
- Atopic dermatitis is a common disease, occurring in up to 7% of children. Approximately 60% of patients with atopic dermatitis develop it in the first year of life; 30% develop it between the ages of 1 and 5. A family history of allergies, asthma, eczema, or hay fever is present in 30 to 70% of patients. Atopic dermatitis is usually worse in the winter.

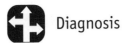 Diagnosis

QUESTIONS THE DOCTOR MAY ASK

- Excessive dryness can worsen dermatitis; the doctor may ask about bathing habits, frequency, and the use of emollients.
- What kind of soap do you use?
- Any contact with new detergents?
- Exposure to new rugs, chemicals, foods?
- A history of skin or allergy problems in the family?
- Possible sources of allergic reaction?

WHAT THE DOCTOR LOOKS FOR

- Examination of the skin

TESTS AND PROCEDURES

- The patch test, if allergies are suspected
- Biopsy or culture of skin may be done.

Dermatitis

 Treatment

GENERAL MEASURES

- For contact dermatitis, mainstay therapy is eliminating future exposure to the irritant or allergen.
- Cool compresses may help contact dermatitis.
- There is no cure for atopic dermatitis. It is a chronic disease with intermittent flares; control is the aim of treatment. Good skin care is critical to maintenance and includes mild soaps, frequent use of emollients, and avoidance of excessive bathing.
- Avoidance of environmental irritants, such as wool sweaters or blankets, is recommended for those with atopic dermatitis. Protective clothing at night to avoid scratching while sleeping is also helpful, as is trimming the nails.
- In infants, seborrhea commonly affects the scalp and responds to frequent use of sulfur or salicylic acid shampoo. If particularly thick, the scales can be loosened first with warm mineral oil or petrolatum, and then gently scrubbed.
- Cradle cap lesions resistant to treatment may respond to a topical steroid lotion rubbed into the scalp with the fingertips.
- Adolescents should use shampoos with zinc pyrithione (Head and Shoulders), selenium sulfide (Selsun), or tar.

ACTIVITY

N/A

DIET

N/A

 Medications

COMMONLY PRESCRIBED DRUGS

- Individuals with seborrheic dermatitis with reddening and severe itching can consider treatment with topical corticosteroid lotions.
- Antihistamines, such as hydroxyzine or diphenhydramine, help to decrease itching of atopic dermatitis.
- Topical anti-itch lotions such as calamine can be helpful for contact dermatitis. This should be applied as moist as possible. The water in calamine is very soothing. Topical corticosteroids and systemic antihistamines help with the itching but do not accelerate resolution of the rash.

Follow-Up

WHAT TO EXPECT

- Atopic dermatitis is a chronic disease. Good skin care is necessary to control disease activity. Up to 40 to 50% of children outgrow their atopic dermatitis after the age of 5.
- Therapy for contact dermatitis should be continued for as long as the rash is present.
- Recovery from contact dermatitis depends on the severity of the condition, but generally improvement is seen in 5 to 7 days.
- The rash of contact dermatitis completely resolves after elimination of further exposure to the allergen.
- In seborrheic dermatitis, some improvement should be seen with therapy by 7 to 10 days. Although this dermatitis is usually self-limited in infancy, it often takes months to resolve completely.
- Cradle cap will self-resolve by the end of the first year of life. The adolescent forms may persist through middle age as a chronic skin dermatitis.

SIGNS TO WATCH

Persistence of rash or evidence of bacterial infection (redness, swelling, discharge)

PREVENTION

Learn to recognize offending agent in contact dermatitis—poisoning leaf.

 Common Questions and Answers

Q: Can the fluid from blisters caused by poison ivy spread the rash to other parts of the body?
A: The contents of the poison ivy blisters are not contagious.

Q: Does therapy eliminate cause of seborrheic dermatitis?
A: Treatment does not appear to influence the underlying cause of this disorder (presumably hormonal influence on the sebaceous glands).

Q: Will the child outgrow atopic dermatitis?
A: Up to 40 to 50% of children outgrow their atopic dermatitis after the age of 5. In some patients, however, the disease persists to a variable extent throughout adulthood.

Q: When atopic dermatitis is controlled, is any treatment necessary?
A: Excessive dryness can worsen the disease; therefore, decreased use of soaps and frequent use of emollients is recommended.

Q: Do food hypersensitivities play a role in atopic dermatitis?
A: This is a debated issue. In general, the majority of patients are probably not adversely affected by foods. However, some individuals, particularly those unresponsive to routine therapy, may benefit from screening for food hypersensitivity and a trial of avoidance to any foods that test positive. The most common foods associated with exacerbation when an association can be made are eggs, milk, wheat, soy, peanuts, and fish.

Diabetes Mellitus, Insulin-Dependent (IDDM or Type I)

 Basics

DESCRIPTION

Diabetes mellitus is a disorder of insulin deficiency. Insulin is necessary for shunting glucose, a sugar, into cells. In IDDM, the cells do not receive sufficient glucose, and high levels of glucose remain outside the cells in the bloodstream (hyperglycemia). IDDM requires the regular administration of insulin.

SIGNS AND SYMPTOMS

- Frequent urination
- Severe thirst, frequent drinking
- Excessive eating
- Loss of appetite
- Weight loss
- Fatigue, lethargy
- Muscle cramps
- Irritability and mood swings
- Vision changes, such as blurriness
- Altered school or work performance
- Headaches
- Anxiety attacks
- Chest pain and occasional difficult breathing
- Abdominal discomfort and pain
- Nausea
- Diarrhea or constipation

CAUSES

- Possibly inherited
- Environmental factors (controversial): viruses, diet, toxins, stress

SCOPE

- IDDM is the most common endocrine/metabolic disorder of childhood.
- IDDM occurs in 1 to 2 per 1000 school-aged children, but the incidence increases with age
  - ▶ 1 in 1500 children under the age of 5 are affected
  - ▶ 1 in 350 by age 16
- IDDM is more common in Northern Europeans, less common in Asians and African-Americans.
- Boys and girls are equally affected.
- 516 new cases per 100,000 children are diagnosed each year.

 Diagnosis

QUESTIONS THE DOCTOR MAY ASK

- Frequent urination, urination during sleep hours, bed-wetting?
- Excessive drinking or eating?
- Weight loss, poor growth?
- Malaise, weakness?
- Changes in behavior, school performance?

WHAT THE DOCTOR LOOKS FOR

- Physical examination
  - Slow-healing skin infection
  - Infection, especially skin and nail-beds
  - Thyroid gland
  - Eye examination

TESTS AND PROCEDURES

- Blood tests (glucose tolerance test)
- Urinalysis

Diabetes Mellitus, Insulin-Dependent (IDDM or TYPE I)

 Treatment

GENERAL MEASURES

- Adequate calories to allow normal growth
- Family education
- Change some activities
- Home monitoring
  - ▶ Checking blood sugar levels
  - ▶ Checking urine for ketones

ACTIVITY

Regular exercise helps to reduce insulin requirements and reduce blood glucose levels.

DIET

- Consistency of amount and timing of meals is important
  - ▶ 20% of daily calories from breakfast and lunch
  - ▶ 30% from dinner
  - ▶ 10% from snacks evenly spaced between meals and before bedtime
- Balance of source of calories is important
  - ▶ 55% from carbohydrates (of which 70% are complex)
  - ▶ 30% from fats
  - ▶ 15% from protein
- American Diabetes Association system of "exchanges" of different food groups
- Carbohydrate "counting"

 Medications

COMMONLY PRESCRIBED DRUGS

Insulin

 Follow-Up

WHAT TO EXPECT

- Regular appointments with diabetologist, nurse specialist, and dietician every 3 months are necessary to assess growth and development and trouble-shoot management problems.
- Meetings with psychologist as needed to address psychosocial and family stressors
- Monitoring of glycosylated hemoglobin every 3 months
- Yearly urine collections
- Yearly ophthalmologic examinations

SIGNS TO WATCH

N/A

PREVENTION

N/A

 Common Questions and Answers

Q: What is the "honeymoon phase"?
A: The period of "remission" after initial stabilization of metabolism with insulin. The honeymoon phase usually lasts weeks to months, but may persist 1–2 years.

Q: What is the risk of diabetes in a sibling or child of a person with type I diabetes?
A: The risk is 2–5% in first-degree relatives (siblings, offspring); 25–35% in identical twins. The risk can be higher in certain cases.

Q: What are the goals of glucose control?
A: Before meals, the blood glucose level should be 80–120 mg/dL. After meals, the blood glucose level should be 180 mg/dL. Additional goals are avoidance of episodes of hypoglycemia (low blood sugar), maintenance of a reasonably nonrestrictive lifestyle, and psychologic adjustment.

Diaper Rash

Basics

DESCRIPTION

Diaper rash, also called diaper dermatitis, is a rash occurring under the covered area of a diaper.

SIGNS AND SYMPTOMS

- Prominent rash on buttocks and pubic skin
- Folds of skin may or may not be affected.
- Genitalia may or may not be affected.
- Child scratches vigorously at night.
- Skin seems chapped.
- May be weeping or crusting
- Swelling

CAUSES

Diaper rashes are the result of several different processes, alone and in combination
- Friction (rubbing of wet diapers against exposed skin areas)
- Irritation
- Allergy
- Seborrhea
- Candidal (yeast) infection

SCOPE

Diaper rash generally resolves when diapers are no longer worn.

Diagnosis

QUESTIONS THE DOCTOR MAY ASK

- Any current medical problems (such as diarrhea)?
- Review skin care techniques: What is put on the skin and how is it used?
- Detergents used in diaper washing?
- Medications used?
- Frequency of diaper changes?
- Crying with urination?
- Almond odor of urine?
- Thrush in mouth?

WHAT THE DOCTOR LOOKS FOR

- Appearance and condition of the affected area
- Any skin disorders at other sites
- Use of medications
- Use of new detergents or soaps

TESTS AND PROCEDURES

Skin may be scraped for microscopic analysis.

Treatment

GENERAL MEASURES

- Proper skin care is the primary treatment.
- When soiled, the skin should be washed gently with a mild soap and patted dry or air-dried.
- The diaper should be kept off and the rash exposed to air as much as possible.
- Topical medication
- Often the caretaker believes the rash is a result of inadequate cleansing of the skin, and subsequently attempts to wash the skin more. This further irritates and worsens the rash. Creams and ointments that strongly adhere to the skin do not need to be scrubbed completely clean before putting on another treatment.
- Nonprescription creams that contain antifungal medications and steroids are often more potent than necessary and can accumulate under the diaper; combination creams are discouraged.
- Talcum powder can worsen the irritation, and may be inhaled by both baby and caretaker. Its use should be discouraged.

ACTIVITY

N/A

DIET

No change in diet is generally necessary.

 ## Medications

COMMONLY PRESCRIBED DRUGS

- Barrier creams, such as zinc oxide, may help protect the skin from external irritants after resolution of the rash.
- If the skin is very inflamed, a small amount of topical corticosteroid cream can be used for a few days.
- Steroid medications should be stopped after a few days, when the intense acute inflammation has improved.
- Topical antifungals: nystatin, miconazole, or clotrimazole for candida
- Topical antifungals should be continued until the rash completely resolves.

 ## Follow-Up

WHAT TO EXPECT

- With proper treatment, the rash should be noticeably better within 4 to 7 days.
- Diaper rash resolves once the child is potty trained and out of diapers.

SIGNS TO WATCH

Failure of resolution of rash indicates that another dermatologic process may be complicating the diaper rash.

 ## Common Questions and Answers

Q: Should I switch from cloth to disposable diapers (or vice versa)?
A: This is debatable, although there are some studies that indicate that the super-absorbent disposable diapers may be better for controlling diaper rashes. Cloth diapers used with plastic overpants probably irritate the skin more because they trap moisture against the skin.

Diarrhea, Acute

Basics

DESCRIPTION

Acute diarrhea, which usually has a rapid onset and is short in duration (less than 2 weeks), is usually caused by intestinal infections. A variety of symptoms are often observed, including frequent passage of loose or watery stools, fever, chills, loss of appetite, vomiting, and malaise. Acute diarrhea can lead to dehydration, failure to thrive, salt imbalances, and other consequences.

- Acute viral diarrhea is the most common form, usually occurs for 1 to 3 days, and is self-limited.
- Bacterial diarrhea develops within 12 hours of eating bacteria-contaminated food.
- Protozoal infections cause prolonged, watery diarrhea that often afflicts travelers returning from areas where the water supply is contaminated.

SIGNS AND SYMPTOMS

- Loose, liquid stools
- Blood or mucus in stool
- Fever
- Abdominal pain and distension
- Headache
- Loss of appetite
- Malaise, fatigue
- Vomiting
- Muscle ache
- Cramping, pale-greasy stools, fatigue, weight loss

SCOPE

- Diarrhea remains one of the most significant global medical problems.
- There are approximately 20 to 40 million episodes of diarrhea in the United States in children less than 5 years of age annually. An estimated 200,000 need hospitalization, and 200–400 die each year.
- Other organisms are transmitted via direct person-to-person contact (day-care centers). Some are transmitted via infected food or water.
- Most common viral organisms occur in the winter months, and the common bacterial organisms occur in the summer.

Diagnosis

QUESTIONS THE DOCTOR MAY ASK

- A careful history needs to be obtained that focuses on possible exposures to other affected individuals, especially children in day-care centers.
- A thorough diet history: how much fluid is ingested
- Antibiotic use
- Travel history
- Stool pattern and symptoms
- Water supply
- Presence of blood in stool
- Unusual odor

WHAT THE DOCTOR LOOKS FOR

- Physical examination
- Evidence of dehydration
- Other sources of fever

TESTS AND PROCEDURES

- Stool culture and analysis
- X-ray of abdomen
- Blood tests—CBC, electrolytes

Treatment

GENERAL MEASURES

- Most cases of acute, infectious diarrhea are mild and self-limited and can be managed on an outpatient basis with close follow-up.
- The goal of therapy is to treat the underlying cause of the diarrhea, if known, and to provide adequate hydration.
- Oral or intravenous fluid replacement therapy may be done.
- The two phases of dehydration correction in patients with acute diarrhea are rehydration and maintenance.
- Antimicrobial agents do not help in most cases.

ACTIVITY

N/A

DIET

Liquids as tolerated, progressing slowly to regular diet

Medications

COMMONLY PRESCRIBED DRUGS

- Oral or intravenous fluids replacement therapy
- When cultures indicate a bacterial infection, antibiodes or other drugs may be used.
- In general, diarrhea medications (immonium) are not helpful and may cause diarrhea stool to remain in intestine.

Follow-Up

WHAT TO EXPECT

- The majority of episodes of acute diarrhea are mild and self-limited. With close supervision and education of hydration status, patients can do very well.
- In more severe cases, close monitoring and reassessment of hydration status is required.
- Once symptoms have improved and the diarrhea has resolved, no routine follow-up is needed.

SIGNS TO WATCH

Dehydration, increasing fever, blood in stool, vomiting that prevents oral hydration

PREVENTION

- The best possible therapy for acute, infectious diarrhea is prevention. The best way to prevent transmission is to interrupt the fecal-oral pathway. For the most part, this requires an increased awareness of sanitation and hygiene as well as the proper handling and cooking of meat, fish, and poultry products.
- Hand washing
- A variety of vaccines are currently being explored.

Common Questions and Answers

Q: How long does the illness last?
A: Typically 3 days for most cases.

Q: What is the most important therapy?
A: Fluids, such as Pedialyte ® Recelyte® or flat ginger ale provide sugar and electrolytes as well as water.

Q: Should food be withheld until diarrhea is gone?
A: After first day of clear fluids, the patient needs calories, so gradual introduction of food is good. Some people use diet of bananas, rice, apples, or toast.

Diarrhea, Chronic

 Basics

DESCRIPTION

Chronic diarrhea lasts for 6 weeks or more. It is less likely than acute diarrhea to be caused by infectious diseases; most commonly it is due to other problems, such as inflammatory bowel disease, malabsorption, or cystic fibrosis.

SIGNS AND SYMPTOMS

- Loose, liquid stools
- Blood or mucus in stool
- Fever
- Abdominal pain and distension
- Headache
- Loss of appetite
- Malaise, fatigue
- Vomiting
- Muscle ache
- Cramping, pale-greasy stools
- Fatigue
- Weight loss

CAUSE

- Salt imbalances
- Intestinal motility disorders
- Inflammation of intestine
- Parasite infection
- Malabsorption

SCOPE

- The various causes of chronic diarrhea change based on the age of the infant. Some are more common in children less than 1 year of age, others in children between 1 and 5 years of age, and others in children older than 5 years of age.
- There is no sex or genetic predisposition that affects the nature of chronic diarrhea.

 Diagnosis

QUESTIONS THE DOCTOR MAY ASK

- The evaluation of a patient with chronic diarrhea needs to begin with a careful and detailed family and dietary history.
- A careful evaluation of the stool pattern, including consistency, frequency, and appearance, must be done.
- The patient's nutritional status and growth parameters need to be studied to determine whether the event is causing malnutrition and/or growth failure.
- Factors that appear to be associated with a worsening or improvement in the diarrhea need to be assessed.

WHAT THE DOCTOR LOOKS FOR

- Physical examination: protuberant abdomen, muscle wasting, dehydration

TESTS AND PROCEDURES

- Stool cultures and analysis
- Blood tests
- Endoscopy and colonoscopy
- Biopsy of intestine

 Treatment

GENERAL MEASURES

- In cases in which infection is detected, appropriate antibiotic therapy should be initiated.
- When there is an offending agent discovered as the cause of the diarrhea, such as cow's milk, soy, lactose, or gluten, these agents should be removed promptly.

- When certain congenital disorders are discovered as the cause of the diarrhea, the therapy is limited and at times only supportive.
- With some causes of chronic diarrhea, a more involved therapy may be indicated. In cases in which tumor, inflammatory bowel disease, or cystic fibrosis is diagnosed, a more chronic and multifactorial treatment regimen needs to be initiated to control the diarrhea and correct the underlying cause.

ACTIVITY

N/A

DIET

- In cases in which there is increased motility and thus increased transit time, such as in chronic nonspecific diarrhea, alterations in the diet can be helpful. Elimination of juices is beneficial. Also, initiating a high-fat, low-carbohydrate diet helps.
- Ensure that the child is getting adequate calories so that his or her nutritional status is not accidentally worsened.
- Avoid the introduction of a regular diet too quickly.

 ## Medications

COMMONLY PRESCRIBED DRUGS

- Antibiotics, if diarrhea is caused by bacterial infection
- Loperamide or Sandostatin®

 ## Follow-Up

WHAT TO EXPECT

- Follow-up for chronic diarrhea varies based on the cause. In cases in which an offending agent is identified and corrected, there is no specific follow-up needed.
- In cases involving congenital defects or immune problems, close observation and adjustment of both medications and nutritional status are needed.
- The time course for improvement and/or resolution of symptoms is based on cause.
- With many of the chronic and complicated causes of chronic diarrhea, the best markers to follow as indicators of disease activity tend to be growth and nutritional status. If the child is able to thrive and grow, the disease is being well-controlled.

SIGNS TO WATCH

Weight gain, change in stool pattern, fever, mouth sores, cough

PREVENTION

N/A

 ## Common Questions and Answers

Q: Why not just use antidiarrhea medicines?
A: It is important to tend the cause and treat that, not just cover up the symptoms.

Q: What is the successful strategy?
A: Many cases are helped by finding the offending food—gluten, certain sugars—and eliminating them from the diet. In other cases, infection can be treated with appropriate medication.

Down Syndrome

 Basics

DESCRIPTION

Down syndrome, also called mongolism or trisomy 21, is a common form of mental retardation. Persons with Down syndrome tend to have many congenital defects, particularly affecting the musculoskeletal system and heart.

SIGNS AND SYMPTOMS

- Typical skull deformity
- Low muscle tone
- Small ears, ear folds, low-set ears
- Mongoloid slant to eyes
- Folds of skin at inner corner of eye
- Depressed nasal bridge
- Enlarged tongue
- Small chin
- Short neck
- Heart murmur
- Dislocated vertebra
- Brushfield spots in iris
- Long crease across entire palm width

CAUSE

Extra or abnormal chromosome 21

SCOPE

- Incidence: 1 of 600–800 live births
- Slightly more common in males
- Risk of Down syndrome increases with maternal age.
- Best recognized and most frequent chromosomal syndrome of humans
- More than 50% of trisomy 21 fetuses are spontaneously aborted in early pregnancy.

 Diagnosis

QUESTIONS THE DOCTOR MAY ASK

- History of infant with Down syndrome in the family?
- Maternal age?
- Fetal movement?

WHAT THE DOCTOR LOOKS FOR

Physical examination, developmental assessment

TESTS AND PROCEDURES

- Prenatal genetic screening
- Fetal ultrasound
- Blood tests of chromosome, thyroid function
- Electrocardiogram (EKG) within the first month of life to rule out cardiac disease; cardiac ultrasound
- Auditory brainstem response within the first 6 months of life
- Echocardiography
- X-rays of head and neck

 Treatment

GENERAL MEASURES

Not applicable except for treatments specific to complications/associated illnesses

ACTIVITY

Have a medical evaluation prior to participation in sports (e.g., Special Olympics).

DIET

N/A

Medications

COMMONLY PRESCRIBED DRUGS

N/A

 ## Follow-Up

WHAT TO EXPECT

- Outcome depends on associated findings.
- As adults, the majority of individuals with Down syndrome can work in supported positions.
- Life expectancy is mildly decreased, with many living into the sixth decade.
- Alzheimer's disease affects approximately 15% of individuals with Down syndrome after the fourth decade of life.

SIGNS TO WATCH

Hearing loss may be misinterpreted as a behavioral problem.

PREVENTION

N/A

 ## Common Questions and Answers

Q: Why was Down syndrome referred to as "mongolism" in the past?
A: There was a mistaken notion about a racial cause for this syndrome because of the facial appearance, which was thought to resemble Mongoloid facial features.

Q: Do all children with Down syndrome have mental retardation?
A: No. Although all persons with Down syndrome have some degree of cognitive disability, some have IQs greater than 70 and are not considered to have mental retardation.

Q: Do children with this syndrome have an increased susceptibility to infection?
A: The literature on this subject is unclear and has been subject to debate. Some children with Down syndrome may have an increased incidence of ear, sinus, and nasolacrimal duct infections. There may be an increased risk of lower respiratory tract infection for children with unrepaired heart disease.

Ear Infection

 ## Basics

DESCRIPTION

Inflammation of the middle ear, or acute otitis media (AOM).

SIGNS AND SYMPTOMS

- Earache
- Fever
- Nasal discharge
- Cough common
- Decreased hearing
- Bleeding or discharge from ear
- Irritability

CAUSES

- Bacterial, viral, or fungal infection
- Normal horizontal position of eustachian tube in infants. This becomes angulated as head grows.

SCOPE

- Highest incidence in children 6 months to 3 years of age
- Higher incidence in boys, Native Americans, Eskimos
- Highest incidence in winter months
- Lower incidence in breastfed infants

 ## Diagnosis

QUESTIONS THE DOCTOR MAY ASK

- Fever?
- Pulling on ear?
- Discharge?
- Hearing loss?
- Medication?

WHAT THE DOCTOR LOOKS FOR

Signs and symptoms of ear infection

TESTS AND PROCEDURES

- Bacterial culture and sensitivity
- Tympanometry: measures middle ear pressures
- Red eardrum
- Fluid in middle ear
- Congenital facial problem

 ## Treatment

GENERAL MEASURES

Antibiotics

ACTIVITY

N/A

DIET

N/A

Medications

COMMONLY PRESCRIBED DRUGS

Antibiotics: Amoxicillin, trimethoprin/sulfa, cefador

 ## Follow-Up

WHAT TO EXPECT

- Improvement within 48 to 72 hours
- Fluid in middle ear may last for 3 months.

SIGNS TO WATCH

- Persistent fever, pain
- Symptoms of complications
- Seriously ill appearance

PREVENTION

- Passive smoke avoidance
- Preventive antibiotics for children with recurrent ear infections

 ## Common Questions and Answers

Q: Are antihistamine/decongestants recommended?
A: Antihistamine/decongestants have not been shown to be effective in the treatment of otitis media and are not recommended.

Encephalitis

 Basics

DESCRIPTION

Encephalitis is an inflammation of the brain.

SIGNS AND SYMPTOMS

- Headache
- Fever
- Malaise
- Stiff neck
- Visual sensitivity to light, lethargy progressing to coma, seizures, neurological deficit
- Progression varies; may be slow or rapid

CAUSE

A direct or delayed reaction by the immune system to a virus, bacteria, fungus, or parasite

SCOPE

- Encephalitis is rare in the United States.
- About 20,000 cases occur annually, most of which are mild.

 Diagnosis

QUESTIONS THE DOCTOR MAY ASK

- Recent viral illness (mono, sore throat)? Rare chicken pox, measles; exposure to herpes virus?
- Recent travel history, pets, and tick bites?
- Travel to area where mosquitos carry virus causing encephalitis

WHAT THE DOCTOR LOOKS FOR

- Physical examination for signs and symptoms of encephalitis
- Neurologic examination

TESTS AND PROCEDURES

- Computed tomography (CT) or magnetic resonance imaging (MRI) of the brain
- Spinal tap, fluid sampled for culture and analysis
- Blood tests
- Viral cultures
- Blood and urine culture
- Toxicology screen
- Electroencephalogram (EEG)

Treatment

GENERAL GUIDELINES

- Patients with encephalitis frequently require intensive care with cardiorespiratory support.
- Early physical and occupational therapies are important.
- Consultation with neurologist, infectious disease specialist, neurosurgeon, and other subspecialists may be helpful.
- Surgery may be required to reduce pressure within the skull.

ACTIVITY

N/A

DIET

N/A

 ## Medications

COMMONLY PRESCRIBED DRUGS

- Antibiotics
- Antiviral drugs
- Antiseizure drugs

 ## Follow-Up

WHAT TO EXPECT

Outcome can range from complete recovery to coma, persistent vegetative state, and death.

SIGNS TO WATCH

N/A

PREVENTION

N/A

 ## Common Questions and Answers

Q: My child has been diagnosed with encephalitis; will he be retarded?
A: The complications after encephalitis vary greatly from severe retardation to full recovery. There is correlation between degree of brain destruction and outcome. However, children frequently recover better than adults with a similar-sized lesion; it is therefore better not to speculate.

Enlarged Breasts (Gynecomastia)

 Basics

DESCRIPTION

Enlarged breasts, or gynecomastia, is an abnormal growth of mammary tissue in males.

SIGNS AND SYMPTOMS

- Increased size of nipples and breast tissue usually occurring at puberty
- Tenderness

CAUSES

- Neonatal gynecomastia
- Gynecomastia of puberty
- Genetic disorder (Klinefelter syndrome)
- Hormone imbalances
- Tumors (pituitary, testicular, adrenal, and liver neoplasms)
- Chronic disease
- Chest nerve trauma or infection, spinal cord lesions
- Drugs

SCOPE

- Vast majority of patients have pubertal gynecomastia.
- Affects 65-80% of pubertal males
- Peak age: 13-15 years

 Diagnosis

QUESTIONS THE DOCTOR MAY ASK

- Medications?
- Tenderness?
- Discharge?
- Timing of onset?
- Degree of gynecomastia?
- Rate of progression?
- Drug exposure?
- Chest wall trauma, surgery, infection?
- Chronic disease?
- Learning disabilities, mental retardation?
- Family history of gynecomastia?

WHAT THE DOCTOR LOOKS FOR

- Physical examination

TESTS AND PROCEDURES

- Usually none
- Blood tests
- Urinalysis
- Genetic screening

Enlarged Breasts (Gynecomastia)

 Treatment

GENERAL MEASURES

- Reassurance
- Elimination or reduction of drugs known to induce gynecomastia, if possible
- Treatment of specific hormonal disorders
- Reexamination at regular intervals (every 3 months initially)
- Cosmetic surgery may be recommended.

ACTIVITY

N/A

DIET

N/A

 Medications

COMMONLY PRESCRIBED DRUGS

Hormonal agents

 Follow-Up

WHAT TO EXPECT

- Spontaneous regression of breast tissue in 6 to 24 months; may be longer
- Overall, prognosis is good.
- Patients with Klinefelter syndrome have a 20-fold increased risk of breast cancer.
- Patients with gynecomastia from other causes are probably also at some increased risk, but breast cancer in these males remains very rare.

SIGNS TO WATCH

- Signs of chronic illness
- Abnormal progression of puberty
- Psychological disorders

 Common Questions and Answers

Q: What causes neonatal gynecomastia?
A: Gynecomastia in newborns is caused by transplacental transfer of estrogens. Galactorrhea also may be present, and resolution generally occurs within a few weeks. Parents should be instructed to refrain from expressing milk as this produces further breast stimulation.

Q: What mechanisms are responsible for drug-induced gynecomastia?
A: Drugs may induce gynecomastia by estrogen-like stimulation (e.g., digitalis, diethlystilbe-strol) or increased estrogen conversion (e.g., phenytoin). Inhibition of testosterone synthesis (e.g., ketoconazole) and increased resistance to testosterone (e.g., cimetidine) are also recognized mechanisms. Hepatic pathways also have been implicated. Often, the mode of stimulation is unknown or may be multifactorial.

Enuresis

 ## Basics

DEFINITION

Enuresis is involuntary urination that occurs after the age of expected bladder control. This term is generally reserved for children 6 years of age or older. In the majority of cases, incontinence occurs only at night (nocturnal enuresis or "bedwetting"). A smaller number of children with enuresis are incontinent during the day, or at both times.

SIGNS AND SYMPTOMS

N/A

CAUSES

- Underlying medical causes are uncommon.
- May be caused by urinary tract infection (UTI)
- Many believe bed-wetting is a delay in development, secondary to smaller bladder capacity.
- Abnormalities of sleep have not been proven to play a role.

SCOPE

- 20% of children have bed-wetting at age 5 years, 10% at age 7 years, 5% at age 10 years, and nocturnal enuresis persists in approximately 1% of adults.
- Daytime wetting occurs in only 1% of 7- to-12-year-olds.
- Bed-wetting is 2–3 times more common in males; daytime wetting is more common in females.
- More common problem among those of lower socioeconomic and educational background

 ## Diagnosis

QUESTIONS THE DOCTOR MAY ASK

- Onset of enuresis
- Nocturnal versus daytime
- The frequency and severity of enuresis
- Pattern of urination: dribbling, painful urination, hesitancy, urgency
- Associated signs and symptoms: stool incontinence, sore muscles, headache, altered consciousness
- History of other medical problems, including urinary tract infections
- Behavior/developmental history: age milestones obtained, toilet training methods, behavioral problems
- Medications
- Effect of enuresis on child: Sleep over with friends or at camp? Teased at school?
- Parents' attitude toward the problem
- Family history of enuresis? If positive, is the child aware?
- Treatments (or punishments) attempted

WHAT THE DOCTOR LOOKS FOR

- Physical examination
- Neurologic examination. Same nerve enervates rectum and bladder, so touching inner buttock area will cause "anal wink". This indicates that nerves to bladder are intact.

TESTS AND PROCEDURES

- Urinalysis
- X-rays of abdomen
- Kidney ultrasound, voiding cystourethrography, renal scan

Treatment

GENERAL GUIDELINES

- Education, reassurance, and support
- Avoid punishment.
- Encourage positive reinforcement: praise, star charts, etc.
- Avoid aggressive therapy in those less than 7 years old.
- Retention training/bladder stretching exercises controversial
- Alarm systems are the most effective of all interventions; several weeks are usually required to achieve complete dryness.

ACTIVITY

N/A

DIET

Fluid restriction in evenings not proven to work

 ## Medications

COMMONLY PRESCRIBED DRUGS

- Desmopressin (DDAVP)
- Imipramine
- Oxybutynin

 ## Follow-Up

WHAT TO EXPECT

- The outcome is very good even without treatment.
- Spontaneous cure rate is 15% per year.

SIGNS TO WATCH

- Social isolation, not wanting to spend night at friend's house

PREVENTION

N/A

 ## Common Questions and Answers

Q: Why do you wait until the child is 5 or 6 to treat?
A: It is so common before that age, we would treat many patients who would stop on their own.

Q: Isn't DDAVP dangerous? What about hyponatremia and volume overload?
A: While the most common side effects noted with DDAVP have been headaches, abdominal pain, and nasal stuffiness, concern remains regarding the potential for hyponatremia and water intoxication. While studies show a safe side effect profile, there have been scattered reports of serious side effects. Use of DDAVP needs to be monitored carefully, especially since it is unclear to what degree variations in aVP levels play in the pathophysiology of PNE.

Q: Won't enuresis recur when DDAVP is stopped?
A: While a significant number of children respond to some degree at the initiation of treatment, results of long-term response to prolonged medication use have varied from study to study. In most instances long-term cure rates have been only slightly better than spontaneous cure rates.

Epiglottitis

 Basics

DESCRIPTION

Epiglottitis is an acute, life-threatening bacterial infection of the epiglottis, a flap of tissue above the larynx, and related structures. It can cause complete airway obstruction, leading to respiratory arrest and death. Epiglottitis constitutes a medical emergency.

SIGNS AND SYMPTOMS

- Develops rapidly
- Fever
- Difficulty swallowing
- Drooling
- Sore throat
- Swollen glands in neck
- Difficulty breathing
- Muffled voice/cry
- Minimal cough
- Shock
- Patient afraid to move

CAUSES

Bacterial infection, typically H. Flu.

SCOPE

- Peaks between 2 and 7 years of age
- Occasional secondary cases in households or day-care centers
- Fortunately, incidence has decreased after immunization for H. Flu (H.b) was instituted.

 Diagnosis

QUESTIONS THE DOCTOR MAY ASK

- History of H.b immunization
- Possibility of swallowing foreign object
- Infectious disease exposure

WHAT THE DOCTOR LOOKS FOR

- Abrupt onset of high fever (greater than 102° F), sore throat, and difficulty swallowing
- Limited or no prodrome
- Rapid onset of toxicity and respiratory distress
- Cough and hoarseness; late symptoms if at all
- Time from onset of symptoms to progressive respiratory distress generally is less than 12 hours.

TESTS AND PROCEDURES

- Blood tests
- Blood culture
- Culture of epiglottis
- X-rays of neck

Therapy

GENERAL MEASURES

- Epiglottitis is a true emergency and requires treatment at a hospital.
- Provide first aid as required, keep airway open, and provide rescue breathing if needed.

ACTIVITY

N/A

DIET

N/A

 ## Medications

COMMONLY PRESCRIBED DRUGS

Antibiotics

 ## Follow-Up

WHAT TO EXPECT

- Death rate is approximately 8%.
- Virtually all fatalities are caused by cardiopulmonary arrest before arrival at the hospital.
- Death rate approaches zero with appropriate airway management.
- Improvement is usually prompt after initiation of appropriate antimicrobial therapy.

SIGNS TO WATCH

- Difficulty swallowing
- Poor air exchange
- Bluish discoloration around eyes, lips, and nail beds
- Lethargy

PREVENTION

- Prevention with rifampin for susceptible children in household, susceptible children in child-care setting, and intimate contacts.
- *Haemophilus influenzae* type b vaccination

 ## Common Questions and Answers

Q: What will the incidence of epiglottitis be in this era of increased early immunization against *H. influenzae* type b?
A: Epiglottitis has already become a rare disease from its previous frequency.

Q: Can epiglottitis recur?
A: Yes, rarely.

Floppy Infant Syndrome

 Basics

DESCRIPTION

Floppy infant syndrome is neuromuscular weakness that typically presents with decreased movement, abnormal posture, or central nervous system dysfunction.

SIGNS AND SYMPTOMS

- Facial weakness (decreased expression)
- Loss of muscle tone
- Abnormal eye movement
- Hip dislocation
- Respiratory problems
- Swallowing/sucking difficulties

CAUSES

- Numerous genetic and metabolic syndromes
- Rare neurologic diseases involving brain, spinal cord, and nerves
- Muscle diseases

SCOPE

Botulism in some cases

 Diagnosis

QUESTIONS THE DOCTOR MAY ASK

- Fetal movements
- Delivery history
- Infections, recent illnesses, and medications
- Family history
- Motor milestone achievement
- Evaluation of mental status

WHAT THE DOCTOR LOOKS FOR

- Physical examination: muscle tone, reflexes, twitching of tongue, drooping eyelids
- Neurologic examination

TESTS AND PROCEDURES

- Blood tests
- Urinalysis
- Electromyography (EMG), nerve conduction velocity (NCV)
- Stool analysis
- Spinal tap
- Magnetic resonance imaging (MRI) or computed tomography (CT)

Treatment

GENERAL MEASURES

- Acute respiratory distress must be anticipated.
- Sucking and swallowing difficulties may necessitate nutritional support.
- Underlying toxic or metabolic causes should be addressed and treated appropriately.
- In many cases, treatment is primarily supportive.
- Orthopedic consultation

ACTIVITY

Physical therapy may be beneficial.

DIET

N/A

 ## Follow-Up

WHAT TO EXPECT

- Developmental milestones and early intervention need to be monitored closely.
- Recovery depends on the cause of weakness.

SIGNS TO WATCH

Respiratory failure, feeding difficulties, developmental milestones

PREVENTION

N/A

 ## Common Questions and Answers

Q: What is Werdnig-Hoffman disease?
A: A disease of the anterior horn cells in the spinal cord; also called infantile spinal muscle atrophy. The earlier the onset of weakness, the poorer the prognosis.

Q: By what age should one expect resolution of benign congenital hypotonia?
A: Hypotonia should not be evident by the time the infant is walking; delay in walking beyond 15 months casts doubt on the diagnosis.

Q: When and how should spinal muscular atrophy (SMA) be ruled out?
A: SMA is a consideration in any infant with insidious onset of significant weakness with arreflexia. Electrophysiologic and (muscle) pathology findings are usually definitive.

Flu

 ## Basics

DESCRIPTION

Influenza, or flu, is an acute, usually self-limited illness caused by an influenza virus. It is marked by fever, inflammation of the nose, throat, eyes, and respiratory tract; and gastrointestinal and systemic symptoms. Outbreaks occur almost every winter with varying degrees of severity. Approximately 10% of children with flu develop pneumonia or other secondary bacterial infections.

SIGNS AND SYMPTOMS

- Abrupt onset of illness beginning with dry cough, runny nose
- Fever, headache, loss of appetite, malaise, muscle ache, sore throat
- Respiratory problems range from mild cough to severe respiratory distress (infants).
- Gastrointestinal problems in younger children may include vomiting (common), diarrhea (uncommon), and severe abdominal pain.

CAUSES

Influenza virus is transmitted from person to person, usually by an airborne route.

SCOPE

- There are 250,000–500,000 new cases of influenza each year.
- Attack rates in healthy children are 10–40% each year.
- Although influenza affects persons of all ages, the most complications and highest mortality rates occur in infants and the elderly.
- Epidemics of influenza occur almost exclusively during winter months.
- Transmission of influenza virus occurs by aerosol droplets and by direct or indirect contact.

 ## Diagnosis

QUESTIONS THE DOCTOR MAY ASK

- Fever?
- Cough?
- Muscle aches?
- Red eyes?
- Diarrhea?

WHAT THE DOCTOR LOOKS FOR

- Infection with the influenza virus causes a distinct set of symptoms.
- Infants and young children may suffer higher fevers and more severe respiratory symptoms.
- Many older children and adults infected with influenza are diagnosed with a "viral respiratory infection," without specific reference to the causative viral agent.
- Associated illnesses include sore throat, croup, bronchitis, bronchiolitis, pneumonia, gastroenteritis, and conjunctivitis (pink eye).

TESTS AND PROCEDURES

- Viral culture
- Rapid tests, polymerase chain reaction (PCR)
- Blood tests
- Chest X-ray

 ## Treatment

GENERAL MEASURES

- Most patients with influenza infection require supportive oral hydration, antifever care, and routine decongestant therapy.
- Anticough medications should be used cautiously and should be appropriate to the age of the child.
- With the exception of the young infant, previously healthy children with influenza infection rarely require emergency treatment.
- Humidified air is helpful to most patients with respiratory symptoms of influenza.
- Respiratory therapy, including endotracheal intubation, may be required for severe cases.
- Intravenous (IV) fluids and supplemental oxygen may be given.

- Patients considered to be at *high risk* for severe disease include those with asthma or other chronic lung disease, severe heart disease, children with a suppressed immune system, and persons traveling to areas where an influenza outbreak is presently occurring.
- Patients considered at *possible high risk* for severe manifestations of influenza include those with HIV infection, sickle cell anemia, diabetes mellitus, chronic kidney disease, chronic metabolic disease, and persons over age 65.
- Patients considered likely to dangerously transmit influenza infection include hospital personnel, especially if there is contact with children or any high-risk patients; household contacts of high-risk patients, including those with HIV; and persons residing in dormitories or other institutional settings.
- Infection with influenza virus may make asthma worse.

ACTIVITY

N/A

DIET

N/A

Medications

COMMONLY PRESCRIBED DRUGS

- Acetaminophen
- Ibuprofen
- Amantadine
- Ribavirin

Follow-Up

WHAT TO EXPECT

- Fever usually lasts up to 5 days.
- Cough may last up to 1 week.
- Lethargy or malaise may persist for up to 2 weeks.

SIGNS TO WATCH

- Signs of secondary bacterial infection
- Rapidly deteriorating mental status or breathing

PREVENTION

- Annual vaccination should be given to high-risk individuals and persons likely to transmit influenza infection to high-risk individuals.
- Children who are receiving chronic aspirin therapy should be considered for vaccination because of the associations between aspirin use, influenza infection, and Reye's syndrome.
- Preventive administration of amantadine is recommended for high-risk children and other subgroups of patients.

Common Questions and Answers

Q: When is it safe for a child with influenza to return to day care or school?
A: Older children with influenza may shed the virus in nasal secretions for up to 7 days from onset of symptoms, younger children even longer. Therefore, older children with influenza may return to school 1 week after the onset of symptoms, and infants and toddlers should remain home for 10-14 days.

Q: Can a child on chronic steroid therapy be immunized against influenza?
A: In general, children who require maintenance steroid therapy for their underlying illness should still receive influenza immunization. If possible, the child should be immunized while on the lowest possible dose of steroids and not during a period of high-dose therapy.

Q: What are the chances of acquiring influenza despite annual vaccination?
A: Vaccination against influenza is greater than 70% effective in preventing disease and greater than 90% effective in preventing death from the infection.

Food Allergy

 Basics

DESCRIPTION

Food allergy is a hypersensitivity reaction caused by certain foods.

SIGNS AND SYMPTOMS

- Gastrointestinal: nausea, vomiting, diarrhea, abdominal pain, flatulence, bloating
- Dermatologic: hives, rash, swelling, dermatitis, pallor, flushing
- Respiratory: runny nose, asthma, cough, earache
- Neurologic: fatigue, fainting, headache
- Other symptoms: systemic reaction, growth retardation, bed-wetting

CAUSES

- Any food or ingested substance can cause allergic reactions. The most commonly implicated foods include cow's milk, egg whites, wheat, soy, peanut, fish, tree nuts (walnut and pecan), shellfish, melons, sesame seeds, sunflower seeds, and chocolate.
- Several food dyes and additives can cause allergic-like reactions.

SCOPE

- The incidence of food allergy ranges from 1 to 7% of the population.
- In children up to 4 years of age, the incidence is between 8 to 16%.
- Only approximately 3–4% of children over 4 years of age have persisting food allergy.

 Diagnosis

WHAT THE DOCTOR LOOKS FOR

- The doctor will take a careful history and do a thorough physical examination to rule out other causes of symptoms.
- The gastrointestinal, dermatologic, respiratory, neurologic, or other signs and symptoms can mimic a variety of diseases.

TESTS AND PROCEDURES

- Blood tests
- Allergy tests: prick test, challenge test
- Analysis of stool
- Abdominal X-rays

Food Allergy

 Treatment

GENERAL MEASURES

- Avoiding the offending food is the most effective way to manage food allergy.
- Individuals with exquisite and severe allergy should carry epinephrine for self-administration in the event that the offending food is ingested unknowingly and a severe reaction develops immediately.
- The success of immunotherapy and hyposensitization has not been proven.

ACTIVITY

N/A

DIET

Avoid foods that cause allergies.

 Medications

COMMONLY PRESCRIBED DRUGS

Diphenhydramine (Benadryl)

 Follow-Up

WHAT TO EXPECT

- A prolonged elimination diet is usually not necessary.
- Tolerance to allergens usually develops by the age of 3.
- Even children with a history of severe allergic reactions most likely outgrow them.
- Reintroduction of foods that trigger allergies should be done under controlled conditions with medical supervision.

SIGNS TO WATCH

N/A

PREVENTION

Avoid triggers.

 Common Questions and Answers

Q: What foods are more likely to be linked to food reactions?
A: Egg, milk, peanut, soy, nuts, wheat, fish, chocolate, and corn.

Food Poisoning

 ## Basics

DESCRIPTION

Food poisoning is an illness caused by food that has been improperly cooked or stored, allowing bacteria to grow. About 40% of food poisoning cases are caused by salmonella, which can cause a broad spectrum of disease states. 25% are caused by staphlococcal infections. Other forms of food poisoning, such as botulism, are the result of powerful toxins produced by bacteria. Typically, food poisoning is marked by a rapid onset of diarrhea, vomiting, and fever 12–72 hours after consuming contaminated food.

SIGNS AND SYMPTOMS

- Nausea, vomiting, diarrhea
- Abdominal cramps
- Bloody diarrhea
- Headache, muscle pain
- Fever to 102°F (39°C); may be persistent
- Bone or joint inflammation
- Wound infection
- Inflammation of heart or blood vessels
- Pneumonia
- Shock
- Urinary tract infection

CAUSES

Contamination by bacteria, resulting from improper cooking or storage of food

SCOPE

- There are about 55 outbreaks of salmonella infections reported annually in the United States. Peak frequency occurs in July to November.
- Children under 5 years old and the elderly are most at risk for salmonella.

 ## Diagnosis

QUESTIONS THE DOCTOR MAY ASK

- Food ingested at picnic in warm weather?
- Other people with similar symptoms?
- Relationship of time of last meal and onset of symptoms?
- Any unusual foods?
- Ingestion of honey (botulism)?
- Handling of chicken prior to cooking?

WHAT THE DOCTOR LOOKS FOR

- Exposure to potential sources of food poisoning
- Physical examination
- Abdominal tenderness
- Signs of dehydration

TESTS AND PROCEDURES

- Stool examination, culture
- Blood tests, blood culture
- Bone marrow sample
- Urine culture
- Other cultures or biopsy

Treatment

GENERAL MEASURES

- Supportive care: maintain proper fluid and salt balances.
- Reduce fever, give pain reliever as needed
- Do not administer antidiarrheal agents.
- Antibiotics may or may not be prescribed.
- Surgery may be necessary.

ACTIVITY

As tolerated

DIET

Oral rehydration solution during diarrhea phase; advance to normal diet as tolerated.

MEDICATION

COMMONLY PRESCRIBED DRUGS

- Antibiotics
- Steroids
- Pain reliever, antifever remedy

Follow-Up

WHAT TO EXPECT

- Fluid and/or salt imbalance is the most common complication of food poisoning.
- Most healthy persons recover spontaneously.
- Some individuals become chronic carriers, persistently shedding bacteria in the stool.
- The relapse rate of fever may approach 15% of patients.

SIGNS TO WATCH

N/A

PREVENTION

- Personal hygiene and sanitation measures are the primary means by which to prevent Salmonella infections.
- Carriers of Salmonella are a public health concern.
- Make sure foods are thoroughly cooked.
- Keep leftovers well-chilled.
- Be careful of cross-contamination by cutting board or utensils; thoroughly wash all utensils and surfaces used to prepare raw foods, especially meat and poultry.

Common Questions and Answers

Q: What are the most common causes of food poisoning?
A: Bacteria (*Salmonella, Staphylococcus*).

Q: How are the signs and symptoms of food poisoning different from a viral gastroenteritis?
A: The signs and symptoms of food poisoning and gastroenteritis are similar in that the patient displays diarrhea, vomiting, and fever. Usually, food poisoning occurs after ingestion of a meal, at which time several people can be affected.

Q: Which foods are most likely to be contaminated?
A: Dairy products that are not refrigerated properly and meat that is not cooked at high enough temperatures.

Frostbite

 ## Basics

DESCRIPTION

Frostbite is damage to skin and subcutaneous tissue from cold exposure and subsequent rewarming; it usually requires temperature below 2°C (36°F).

SIGNS AND SYMPTOMS

- Superficial, first-degree: white and waxy skin while frozen; then reddening, swelling, and sensation of heat. Stinging and burning followed by throbbing and aching. Skin may peel 5–10 days later.
- Superficial, second-degree: white and waxy while frozen; then reddening, substantial swelling, and blister formation. Skin death occurs 5–10 days later.
- Deep, third-degree: Fluid or blood-filled blisters form over 3 days to a week. Skin death and blue-gray discoloration occur in 5–10 days. No sensation initially; skin feels like "block of wood." Later, burning, aching, throbbing, and shooting pains are felt.

CAUSE

- Exposure to cold
- Circulatory problems

SCOPE

Various groups are at increased risk of frostbite:
- Homeless or malnourished children
- Those with altered mental status, such as adolescents with psychiatric disorders and children/adolescents using drugs or alcohol
- Those engaged in outdoor play/sports, especially skiing, running, mountain climbing; also seen in urban settings with games such as winter football
- Older adolescents exposed to cold in military or on the job

 ## Diagnosis

QUESTIONS THE DOCTOR MAY ASK

- Treatments tried?
- Rubbing snow?
- Hot water?

WHAT THE DOCTOR LOOKS FOR

- Prolonged exposure to cold weather
- Short exposure to extreme cold (e.g., touching cold metal causes immediate frostbite)
- Timing of exposure
- Fingers, toes, nose, and ears (unprotected, distal extremities) most often affected

 ## Treatment

GENERAL MEASURES

- Hypothermia usually is managed at a hospital emergency department or intensive care unit.
- Provide emergency first aid as needed, including rescue breathing and cardiopulmonary resuscitation.
- Remove wet garments.
- Protect against heat loss and wind chill.
- Maintain horizontal position.
- Move victim to a warm location as quickly as possible; alert 9-1-1.
- Surgery may be required.

ACTIVITY

N/A

DIET

N/A

Medications

COMMONLY PRESCRIBED DRUGS

- Antibiotics
- Ibuprofen

 ## Follow-Up

WHAT TO EXPECT

- Superficial first-degree frostbite may heal within 2 weeks.
- Deep frostbite may take months for spontaneous healing to be completed.
- Cold sensitivity, damp skin, and changes in skin color are common, long-lasting complications.

SIGNS TO WATCH

N/A

PREVENTION

- Public education addressing how to dress appropriately for outdoor winter activities and advising when the weather risk is greatest
- Nicotine has vasoconstrictive properties; *smoking should not be permitted.*

 ## Common Questions and Answers

Q: How can I prevent my child from getting frostbite while he or she plays outdoors in the winter?
A: Dress the child in multiple layers of clothing. Use waterproof clothing as the outer layer, especially gloves and boots. Cover nose and ears well. Encourage frequent breaks to come indoors, check for frostbite, and rewarm. Do not let the child return outdoors if there is evidence of even mild frostbite. Encourage indoor play in extremes of weather, including high winds.

Q: My child had frostbite in the past. Do I need to take special precautions with him?
A: Yes. Your child is much more likely to have frostbite again in the previously affected area. You need to be especially vigilant with dress, and remove the child from cold conditions sooner than one might otherwise.

Q: How will I know if my child has frostbite rather than just cold fingers?
A: Cold fingers usually look red, while fingers with frostbite look white and waxy before rewarming. If the fingers are placed in warm water, they then turn red. In either case, warm with warm water, not dry heat.

Fungal Infection

 Basics

DESCRIPTION

Superficial fungal infections often involve the skin, hair, or nails. Common fungal infections include tinea, ringworm, athlete's foot, and candidiasis.

SIGNS AND SYMPTOMS

- Onset may be sudden (as in the case of a diaper rash), but usually the skin changes gradually (e.g., the characteristic ring of "ringworm").
- Usually itchy
- Ringworm:
  - ▶ Round, ring-shaped lesion on skin
  - ▶ Mildly reddened and flaky
  - ▶ Appearance may vary depending on degree of inflammation.
- Candidiasis:
  - ▶ Reddened, often fiery
  - ▶ Satellite lesions
  - ▶ Usually itchy
  - ▶ Favors skin folds/creases (armpits, groin, below the breasts, and, in infants, the diaper area)
- Tinea versicolor:
  - ▶ Oval patches of scaly skin
  - ▶ Distribution typically over shoulders, neck, and back, occasionally occurs on face
  - ▶ Skin often has altered pigmentation, either increased or decreased.

CAUSES

Variety of fungi, including dermatophytes (ringworm), trichophyton—skin and hair, and candida

SCOPE

Fungal infections are common.

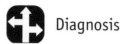 **Diagnosis**

QUESTIONS THE DOCTOR MAY ASK

- Travel or pet exposure, especially contact with stray cats?
- Other family members infected?

WHAT THE DOCTOR LOOKS FOR

Examines the nature, extent, and severity of skin disorder

TESTS AND PROCEDURES

- Skin may be scraped for laboratory analysis.
- Fungal culture
- Wood-lamp examination

 Treatment

GENERAL MEASURES

- Proper hygiene
- Careful hand-washing
- Launder towel, clothing, and head wear of infected individual.
- Check other family members.
- Topical medications

ACTIVITY

N/A

DIET

N/A

Medications

COMMONLY PRESCRIBED DRUGS

- Griseofulvin
- Itraconazole
- Imidazole
- Terbinifine
- Nystatin
- Selenium sulfide

Follow-Up

WHAT TO EXPECT

- Lesions may take weeks to clear, but the inflammation should begin to improve within several days.
- Candidal skin lesions usually improve within 24 to 48 hours and resolve by 5 to 7 days.
- Relapses and recurrences are common.

SIGNS TO WATCH

- Watch the surrounding area for signs of bacterial infection, such as reddening or drainage.
- Highly inflamed lesions that do not improve within the first few days may require a course of oral steroids.

PREVENTION

- Children should be discouraged from sharing clothing, especially hats, with others.
- Pets should be watched and treated early for any suspicious lesions.
- Avoid risk factors.
- Avoid contact with suspicious lesions.
- Maintain good personal hygiene.
- Wear rubber or wooden sandals in community showers or bathing places.
- Carefully dry between the toes after showering or bathing.
- Change socks frequently.
- Apply drying or dusting powder.

Common Questions and Answers

Q: How is the management of a child with both scalp and body ringworm different from the child with a body lesion alone?
A: Scalp lesions must be treated with an oral agent (e.g., griseofulvin) to eliminate the fungus from the hair follicle.

Gastritis

 ## Basics

DESCRIPTION

Gastritis is an inflammation of the lining of the stomach. Gastritis is the most common cause of upper gastrointestinal tract bleeding in children.

SIGNS AND SYMPTOMS

- Upper abdominal pain, usually after meals
- Loss of appetite
- Vomiting after meals
- Irritability
- Poor feeding and weight loss
- Less often: chest pain, vomiting blood, or dark tarry stools

CAUSES

- Infection (e.g., tuberculosis, *Helicobacter pylori*, cytomegalovirus, parasites)
- Stress
- Unknown
- Caustic ingestions (e.g., lye, strong acids, pine oil)
- Drug-induced (e.g., nonsteroidal anti-inflammatory drugs [NSAIDS], steroids, valproate)
- Alcohol consumption
- Protein sensitivity (e.g., cow's milk protein allergy)

SCOPE

Gastritis is one of the most common gastrointestinal diagnoses in children.

 ## Diagnosis

QUESTIONS THE DOCTOR MAY ASK

- Pain?
- Vomiting?
- Irritability?
- Poor feeding?

WHAT THE DOCTOR LOOKS FOR

Signs and symptoms of gastritis—abdominal tenderness

TESTS AND PROCEDURES

- Stool test for blood
- Blood tests
- Upper gastrointestinal (GI) series
- Endoscopy
- Culture of gastric biopsy

 ## Treatment

GENERAL MEASURES

- Supportive care with close monitoring of intake and output
- Mental status

ACTIVITY

N/A

DIET

Dietary changes not helpful

Medications

COMMONLY PRESCRIBED DRUGS

- Antacids or H_2 blockers
  - ▶ Ranitidine
  - ▶ Cimetidine
  - ▶ Famotidine
  - ▶ Omeprazole
- Discontinue NSAIDS
- Eliminate alcohol and tobacco
- If symptoms persist: antibiotics, bismuth

 ## Follow-Up

WHAT TO EXPECT

- Repeat blood tests
- Endoscopy may be repeated.

SIGNS TO WATCH

- Monitor for blood in stools.
- Antacids are not palatable to children and can lead to diarrhea or constipation.

PREVENTION

N/A

 ## Common Questions and Answers

Q: Will a bland diet help gastritis to resolve?
A: Dietary changes have not been shown to affect the natural course of gastritis.

Q: What is *H. pylori?*
A: *H. pylori* is a bacterium frequently found in the stomachs of patients with gastritis and peptic ulcer disease. *H. pylori* infection is diagnosed with special tests and is treated with antibiotics. Relapse rates for gastritis caused by *H. pylori,* however, are high.

Gastroesophageal Reflux

 Basics

DESCRIPTION

Gastroesophageal reflux (GER) disease is the effortless regurgitation of the stomach contents into the esophagus, which can cause irritation or inflammation of the esophagus. The disorder is common in infants. Most episodes are brief and cause no symptoms. GER is associated with irritability, pain, inflammation or bleeding of the esophagus, failure to thrive, asthma, near-miss SIDS, and pneumonia. GER may not cause symptoms and still carry the risk of complications.

SIGNS AND SYMPTOMS

- Vomiting
- Failure to thrive
- Breathing difficulty
- Sleep apnea
- Difficulty swallowing
- Asthma
- Cough

CAUSE

- Disorder of stomach muscle
- Other gastric disorders

SCOPE

GER is the most common cause of vomiting in infancy.

 Diagnosis

QUESTIONS THE DOCTOR MAY ASK

- Family history of metabolic disease?
- Family history of allergies?
- Position of baby after feeding?
- Weight gain or loss?
- Presence of cough?

WHAT THE DOCTOR LOOKS FOR

- Signs and symptoms of gastroesophageal reflux
- Episodes of near-miss SIDS, pneumonia, chronic cough, laryngitis, noisy breathing, and asthma
- Infection, metabolic disease, allergy, and neurologic disease must be ruled out.
- Growth failure, blood in the stool, asthma, anemia, or other signs may suggest complications.

TESTS AND PROCEDURES

- Stool analysis
- Growth parameters
- Upper gastrointestinal (GI) series
- Chest X-ray
- Nuclear medicine studies
- pH probe
- Endoscopy
- Digestive system pressure studies

Treatment

GENERAL MEASURES

- Several modes of therapy are available, depending on the severity, duration of reflux, and complications.
- The treatment should be individualized.
- Small, frequent feedings
- Thickening of the feedings (approximately 1 tablespoon cereal per ounce of formula)
- Positioning: Use infant seat for 2 to 3 hours after meals.
- A hypoallergenic formula may be recommended for children with associated food allergy.
- Surgery may be recommended.

ACTIVITY

N/A

DIET

- Small, frequent feedings
- Thickening

 ## Medications

COMMONLY PRESCRIBED DRUGS

- Antacids
- Cisapride (Propulsid)
- Metaclopramide (Reglan)
- Cimetidine (Tagamet)
- Ranitidine (Zantac)
- Famotidine (Pepcid)
- Omeprazole (Prilosec)
- Sucralfate (Carafate)

 ## Follow-Up

WHAT TO EXPECT

Most infants eventually outgrow the symptoms.

SIGNS TO WATCH

Growth pattern, onset of cough

 ## Common Questions and Answers

Q: What are indications for surgery?
A: Poor response to medicine management.

Q: What are complications of surgery?
A: Vomiting, obstruction, feeding difficulty, recurrence of reflux.

German Measles

 ## Basics

DESCRIPTION

German measles, or rubella, is a viral infection characterized by mild symptoms with a red rash progressing from head to toes. Infection of a woman during pregnancy can cause birth defects.

SIGNS AND SYMPTOMS

- In adults, a 1- to 5-day episode of low-grade fever, malaise, and enlarged neck glands may precede the rash.
- The rash begins on the face, then progresses to the trunk and extremities. The rash usually lasts for 3 days.
- Enlarged lymph nodes
- Joint pain, arthritis in adults

CAUSE

Rubella virus

SCOPE

Currently, fewer than 1000 cases per year are reported.

 ## Diagnosis

QUESTIONS THE DOCTOR MAY ASK

- History of rubella immunization (MMR)?
- Exposure?
- Contact with pregnant women?

WHAT THE DOCTOR LOOKS FOR

Signs and symptoms of German measles
- Rash
- Lymph node behind ear
- Red eyes

TESTS AND PROCEDURES

- Viral isolation from throat or urine
- Blood tests

 ## Treatment

GENERAL MEASURES

Supportive care

ACTIVITY

Individuals who are infectious should avoid pregnant females.

DIET

N/A

Follow-Up

WHAT TO EXPECT

- The prognosis is good. As many as 50% of infections cause no symptoms.
- Rubella infection in a pregnant woman can cause severe birth defects in the infant.

SIGNS TO WATCH

N/A

PREVENTION

Vaccination

 Common Questions and Answers

Q: While pregnancy is a contraindication to rubella vaccination, if a pregnant woman is inadvertently vaccinated, will there be harm to the fetus?

A: There is no evidence of harm to women who were vaccinated while pregnant.

Glucose-6-Phosphate Dehydrogenase (G6PD) Deficiency

 ## Basics

DESCRIPTION

Deficiency of the enzyme glucose-6-phosphate dehydrogenase (G6PD) can result in hemolytic anemia. Anemia may be mild or severe, leading to kidney failure and the need for transfusion.

- Individuals deficient in G6PD are generally free of symptoms, but may have episodes of acute anemia resulting from stressors such as drugs or infections.
- Favism, or anemia related to fava bean ingestion, is always caused by G6PD deficiency, but not all deficient patients develop this condition.

SIGNS AND SYMPTOMS

- History of recent infection
- Pallor
- Jaundice
- Rapid heart rate
- Fatigue, malaise
- Dark urine
- Family history of jaundice or G6PD deficiency
- Bleeding (which may not be obvious)

CAUSE

Genetic defect

SCOPE

- It is the most common of all clinically significant enzyme defects.
- Over 400 variants have been discovered and named.

 ## Diagnosis

QUESTIONS THE DOCTOR MAY ASK

New medications, fava bean consumption, recent or current illnesses, and previous similar episodes? Family history of anemia? Fatigue, malaise?

WHAT THE DOCTOR LOOKS FOR

Signs and symptoms of hemolytic anemia: paleness, presence of enlarged spleen

TESTS AND PROCEDURES

- Blood tests
- Genetic screening

 ## Treatment

GENERAL MEASURES

- Remove stressor: Discontinue suspected drug and/or treat infection.
- Transfusion is rarely necessary.
- Supportive care, evaluation of kidney, and monitoring degree of anemia are important.
- Education regarding drug avoidance, signs and symptoms of hemolysis, and family and genetic counseling should be provided.

ACTIVITY

N/A

DIET

Avoid fava beans.

Glucose-6-Phosphate Dehydrogenase (G6PD) Deficiency

 Follow-Up

WHAT TO EXPECT

- Most individuals with G6PD deficiency are free of symptoms.
- When hemolysis does occur, it tends to be self-limited and resolves spontaneously with a return to normal levels in 2 to 6 weeks.
- The development of kidney failure is extremely rare in children.

SIGNS TO WATCH

See signs and symptoms

PREVENTION

N/A

 Common Questions and Answers

Q: Do I need to follow a special diet or avoid medications if I have G6PD deficiency?
A: Although most patients have no symptoms of their disease, certain medications may cause transient anemia, and these drugs should be avoided. When prescribing medications, your physician and pharmacist should know about your G6PD deficiency, but most necessary medications are safe and well-tolerated. People with severe variants of the deficiency should also avoid fava beans, but otherwise, no dietary restrictions are necessary.

Q: Do I need to know which variant of G6PD deficiency I have?
A: It may be clear which variant you are likely to have based on your clinical symptoms and ethnic background. In most cases, it is unnecessary to do biochemical testing, except in more severe cases or when the diagnosis is uncertain.

Q: Should my family be screened if someone has G6PD deficiency?
A: Population screening is generally not necessary unless there is a strong ethnic prevalence of a severe variant.

Goiter

 Basics

DESCRIPTION

Goiter is the enlargement of the thyroid gland.

SIGNS AND SYMPTOMS

- Enlargement, swelling, or lump on neck
- Pain, difficulty swallowing
- Hyperthyroidism: hyperactivity, irritability, excessive eating, weight loss
- Hypothyroidism: sedentary, quiet, gaining weight, constipation

CAUSES

Multiple causes
- Inflammation of thyroid
- Iodine deficiency
- Drugs—lithium, contraceptives

SCOPE

- Prevalence of goiter in the United States is 3–7%.
- In regions of iodine deficiency, the incidence of goiter is much higher.

 Diagnosis

QUESTIONS THE DOCTOR MAY ASK

- School performance?
- Head, neck, or chest radiation?
- Diet?
- Pain?
- Change in size?

WHAT THE DOCTOR LOOKS FOR

History and physical examination should focus on determining whether the child has signs and symptoms of hypothyroidism or hyperthyroidism.

TESTS AND PROCEDURES

- Blood tests
- Ultrasound

Treatment

GENERAL MEASURES

- Therapy is dictated by the cause of the goiter.
- Surgery to decrease the size of a goiter is indicated only if adjacent structures are compressed.

ACTIVITY

N/A

DIET

Depends on the cause of the goiter. The incidence of iodine deficiency (endemic) goiter has greatly declined since the introduction of potassium iodide to salt. Iodide can also be added to communal drinking water or administered as an iodized oil in isolated rural areas.

 ## Medications

COMMONLY PRESCRIBED DRUGS

- L-thyroxine
- Propylthiouracil, methimazole

 ## Follow-Up

WHAT TO EXPECT

- Duration of therapy depends on the cause of the goiter.
- Potential for regression of goiter depends on cause.
- The outcome depends on the cause of the goiter.
- Goiter may or may not decrease in size with treatment.

SIGNS TO WATCH

Thyroid dysfunction, overactivity, heat intolerance, nervousness

 ## Common Questions and Answers

Q: Will the goiter decrease in size with treatment?
A: This depends again on the cause of the goiter. For example, in CLT if an elevated TSH is present, treatment can result in a decrease in size of the goiter. In idodine-deficient states treatment will cause the *early* hyperplastic goiter to regress.

Hand-Foot-and-Mouth Disease

 Basics

DESCRIPTION

Hand-foot-and-mouth disease is a viral illness that causes an outbreak of blistering ulcers around the mouth, a rash of the hands and/or feet, and mild constitutional symptoms, such as fever and malaise.

SIGNS AND SYMPTOMS

- A mild illness occasionally precedes the rash by 1 or 2 days: low-grade fever (usually near 100° F), malaise, sore mouth, loss of appetite, runny nose, diarrhea, abdominal pain
- Oral lesions begin as small, red bumps.
- Quickly evolve to small blisters on a reddened base
- Lesions progress to ulcerations.
- Tongue, cheek, palate, gums, and tonsils may be affected.
- Oral lesions may persist up to 1 week.
- Rash affecting the back of the hands and toes
- Rash may also occur on the palms, soles, arms, legs, buttocks, and face.
- Eruptions progress to blisters.
- Rarely tender or itchy

CAUSES

Viral infection

SCOPE

- In temperate climates, hand-foot-and-mouth disease is most common in the late summer and fall.
- It is spread primarily by fecal contamination and contact. Oral and respiratory secretions may also transmit the virus.
- Incubation period is 3 to 7 days.
- Highly contagious, afflicting up to half of those exposed
- Close household contacts are particularly susceptible.
- May occur as an isolated case or in an epidemic.
- Most common in children under 5 years old, but may affect adults

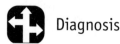 Diagnosis

QUESTIONS THE DOCTOR MAY ASK

- Exposure?
- Bone or joint pain?
- Hydration?
- Urine output?

WHAT THE DOCTOR LOOKS FOR

- The location, type, and severity of skin lesions
- Symptoms of dehydration, encephalitis, pneumonia, inflamed heart, or other complications

TESTS AND PROCEDURES

- Viral culture and identification
- Blood tests

Treatment

GENERAL MEASURES

- Most cases spontaneously resolve and require no therapy other than reassurance.
- Good supportive care is generally sufficient to treat most complications.
- Symptomatic relief from particularly painful oral ulcers may be accomplished by application of a topical antihistamine or anesthetic directly to the sores (see Common questions and answers).
- Dehydration should be treated when present. Intravenous fluids may be required in severe cases of dehydration, especially in infants and young children.

ACTIVITY

N/A

DIET

Dietary adjustments often improve oral intake and prevent or relieve dehydration:
- ▶ Avoid spicy or acidic foods.
- ▶ Provide cool or iced liquids in small quantities frequently.

 Medications

COMMONLY PRESCRIBED DRUGS

Acetaminophen may relieve malaise and minor discomfort associated with the oral ulcers. It also may be used to reduce fever.

 Follow-Up

WHAT TO EXPECT

- Hand-foot-and-mouth disease generally resolves spontaneously within 1 week after diagnosis.
- Small children must be followed closely for signs of dehydration.
- Some patients may become carriers without symptoms.

SIGNS TO WATCH

N/A

PREVENTION

- Frequent hand washing, especially after changing diapers, and good personal hygiene are the most useful means to prevent spread of viral illnesses.
- The period of eruptions and the preceding illness appear to be the most contagious; however, some carriers may shed virus in the stool 3 months after infection.

 Common Questions and Answers

Q: What is in the "magic mouthwash" often used to relieve the pain of oral ulcers?
A: Many health care providers prescribe a "magic mouthwash" for relief of oral ulcers, sore throat, and teething pain. The most common such treatment consists of equal parts of aluminum hydroxide/magnesium hydroxide gel suspension and diphenhydramine elixir (12.5 milligrams per 5 milliliters). It can be applied directly to the sores with a cotton swab or a small syringe before meals.

Q: When may children with hand-foot-and-mouth disease return to school?
A: This is a matter of some controversy for this highly contagious, but relatively benign, condition. On the one hand, good hygiene greatly reduces viral transmission. On the other, affected patients are often contagious before the diagnosis is made. Most doctors now suggest isolation from school or day-care contacts while fever and/or rash persists. As mentioned, some may shed the virus in their stool for months after symptoms have resolved (again stressing the need for good personal hygiene).

Heat Stroke and Exhaustion

 Basics

DESCRIPTION

Heat exhaustion and heat stroke are severe illnesses caused by dehydration, loss of salts, and failure of the body's temperature regulation mechanisms.

- Heat exhaustion is an acute heat injury due to dehydration.
- Heat stroke is extreme injury with failure of temperature regulation that profoundly affects the central nervous system.

SIGNS AND SYMPTOMS

- Heat exhaustion:
  - Weakness, lethargy, thirst, malaise, diminished ability to work or play, headache, nausea, vomiting, muscle ache, pale skin, dizziness, visual disturbances, fainting, mild central nervous system dysfunction, impaired judgment, cramps, dizziness, rapid heart rate, rapid breathing rate, loss of sensation or tingling, agitation, incoordination, psychosis, temperature below 105° F (40°C), sweating
- Heat stroke:
  - Temperature greater than 105°F (40.5°C), with or without hot, dry (classic) or clammy skin; pink or ashen skin; weakness; nausea; vomiting; loss of appetite; headache; dizziness; confusion; drowsiness; irritability; central nervous system dysfunction; euphoria; combativeness; abrupt or impending alteration of consciousness; rapid heart rate; rapid breathing rate; difficulty moving; incontinence; seizures

CAUSES

Failure of heat-dissipating mechanisms or an overwhelming heat stress leading to a rise in core temperature and dehydration and salt depletion

SCOPE

Varies depending on pre-existing conditions and environmental factors

 Diagnosis

QUESTIONS THE DOCTOR MAY ASK

- Cooling maneuvers en route to hospital?
- Initial temperature if taken at scene?
- Any history of central nervous system dysfunction?
- Any predisposing medical, environmental, or activity issues?

WHAT THE DOCTOR LOOKS FOR

- Headache
- Weakness
- Muscle pain
- Cramps
- Disorientation
- Rapid heart rate
- Incoordination

TESTS AND PROCEDURES

- Core body temperature
- Blood tests
- Arterial blood gasses
- Spinal tap
- Chest X-ray
- Electrocardiogram (EKG)

 Treatment

GENERAL MEASURES

- Heat injuries are emergencies that are best managed in a hospital.
- Heat stroke is a life-threatening emergency.
- Remove person to a cooler location.
- Provide emergency first aid as needed (rescue breathing, cardiopulmonary resuscitation [CPR]).
- Rapid cooling: remove clothing, wet patient down, ice packs
- Intravenous fluids
- For heat cramps: rest, salt and water replacement
- For heat fainting: horizontal position, rest, fluids (salted liquids)

Heat Stroke and Exhaustion

ACTIVITY

N/A

DIET

N/A

Medications

COMMONLY PRESCRIBED DRUGS

- Chlorpromazine
- Benzodiazepine

Follow-Up

WHAT TO EXPECT

- Heat illness (heat rash, swelling, cramps, fainting, exhaustion): rapid recovery with supportive care
- Heat stroke: poor prognosis if not recognized and aggressively managed
- Heat stroke mortality rate is 10%.
  - ▸ The mortality rate is related to peak temperature and duration.
  - ▸ With treatment delay of 2 hours, the risk of death is 70%.
- Can have persistent central nervous system dysfunction

SIGNS TO WATCH

See Signs and symptoms

PREVENTION

- Recognize individuals at risk and conditions that predispose to development of heat illness.
- Limit physical activity
- Keep cool during hot, humid weather.
- Use air conditioning all or part of hot days.
- Cool or tepid baths
- Increase fluid intake: unlimited fluid replacement during strenuous activity
- Loose, light-colored clothing
- Acclimatization, gradual conditioning (7–14 days)
- Liberal dietary sodium
- Frequently flex leg muscles when standing and avoid prolonged standing in hot environments.

Common Questions and Answers

Q: How can one distinguish between heat exhaustion and heat stroke?
A: If CNS abnormalities are present, temperature is > 40.6°C and liver function tests are elevated, the patient is likely to have heat stroke. Remember, however, that CNS examination and temperature upon arrival to medical care may not be representative of the maximal abnormalities die to preceding interventions.

Q: When should heat stroke be suspected?
A: Suspect heat stroke in a patient with or without sweating who demonstrates alterations of CNS function in environment that would be conducive to heat illness.

Q: Does the presence or absence of sweating help with the diagnosis of heat exhaustion versus heat stroke?
A: No. Sweating will be present with heat exhaustion and may or may not be present with heat stroke.

Hemolytic Anemia of the Newborn

 Basics

DESCRIPTION

This type of hemolytic anemia occurs in the newborn when mother's cells react with infant's blood and causes destruction of the cells and anemia. It occurs in newborns with Rh-positive blood but whose mothers have Rh-negative blood. During a first pregnancy, the Rh-negative mother may make antibodies to the Rh factor if the fetus is Rh-positive. During a second pregnancy, these Rh antibodies in the mother's bloodstream can cause serious problems in the developing fetus (if it is Rh-positive) and lead to hemolytic anemia.

SIGNS AND SYMPTOMS

- Pallor, rapid heart and breathing rate caused by congestive heart failure (CHF)
- Generalized swelling

CAUSES

Immune system response

SCOPE

Affects 6–7 per 1000 live births

 Diagnosis

QUESTIONS THE DOCTOR MAY ASK

- Mother's blood type?
- Use of RhoGAM if mother is Rh negative?

WHAT THE DOCTOR LOOKS FOR

Signs and symptoms of hemolytic anemia in the newborn

TESTS AND PROCEDURES

- Blood tests
- Amniocentesis during pregnancy
- Fetal blood sampling in severe cases

 Treatment

GENERAL MEASURES

Hospital treatment of newborn

ACTIVITY

N/A

DIET

N/A

Hemolytic Anemia of the Newborn

 Medications

COMMONLY PRESCRIBED DRUGS

Rhogam, for treatment of unsensitized mother at 28 weeks of pregnancy

 Follow-Up

WHAT TO EXPECT

- Approximately one-half the infants have minimal anemia and require no treatment or light therapy only.
- One-fourth require blood transfusions.

SIGNS TO WATCH

N/A

PREVENTION

N/A

 Common Questions and Answers

Q: Does the condition become worse with each pregnancy?
A: Yes, if the mother is not treated with Rh immunoglobulin after each Rh-positive pregnancy or abortion.

Hemophilia

 Basics

DESCRIPTION

Hemophilia is a bleeding disorder caused by the absence, severe deficiency, or defective functioning of blood clotting factors. Factor 8 deficiency—hemophilia A. Factor 9 deficiency—hemophilia B.

SIGNS AND SYMPTOMS

- Spontaneous joint and muscle hemorrhages, easy bruising, and prolonged and potentially fatal bleeding after trauma or surgery
- Excessive bleeding with circumcision or of the umbilical cord may be an initial presentation.
- Bleeding generally occurs with increasing frequency around the time the child begins to walk or starts teething.

CAUSE

Genetic defect X-linked recessive—carried by mother with disease in males.

SCOPE

- Most common severe hereditary clotting disorder
- X-linked genetic disorder, affecting males almost exclusively
- Incidence: 20 per 100,000 male births

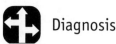 Diagnosis

QUESTIONS THE DOCTOR MAY ASK

History of hemophilia in family?

WHAT THE DOCTOR LOOKS FOR

- Hemophilia is suspected whenever unusual bleeding is encountered in a male patient.
- A family history of hemophilia in male offspring of female blood relatives is present in 30 to 40% of cases.
- No excessive bleeding after minor cuts or abrasions

TESTS AND PROCEDURES

Blood tests, particularly blood coagulation tests

Treatment

GENERAL MEASURES

- Factor replacement
- Immobilization: splints, casts, crutches, and/or bedrest
- Special management is required for major surgery, compartment syndrome, oral bleeding, and special bleeding situations such as intracranial bleeding.
- Suture placement should be avoided when possible.
- Blood in urine: Increased fluid intake and bedrest may be used as an initial treatment.
- If blood persists in urine, factor replacement is necessary.
- Some patients are treated preventively on a regular schedule (e.g., 3 times/week) to prevent bleeding episodes.

ACTIVITY

Avoid aggressive contact sports, e.g., football, basketball, lacrosse, hockey, rugby; tennis and baseball are OK, but the child may be prone to small joint bleeds.

DIET

N/A

 ## Medications

COMMONLY PRESCRIBED DRUGS

- Clotting factor: Factor 8 replacement for hemophilia A; factor 9 replacement for hemophilia B.
- DDAVP

 ## Follow-Up

WHAT TO EXPECT

- Complications of hemophilia:
  - ▸ Hemophilic joint damage and disability from recurrent bleeds characterized by joint contractures, limited range of motion, chronic pain
  - ▸ Intracranial bleeding
  - ▸ Compartment syndrome
  - ▸ Airway compromise due to bleeds in the throat, tongue, or neck
- Five to twenty percent develop antibodies against clotting factors.

SIGNS TO WATCH

N/A

PREVENTION

- Good dental hygiene
- Immunizations: no intramuscular injections; given subcutaneously with a small-gauge needle
- Rapid treatment to avoid chronic joint damage
- Home infusion therapy as appropriate for family
- Self-infusion training: usually start around 11 years of age

 ## Common Questions and Answers

Q: How is this different from bruising?
A: Bruising usually is less severe and will stop with pressure or with no treatment. Tests exist that help differentiate the two problems.

Hernia

 Basics

DESCRIPTION

A hernia is the protrusion of a portion of abdominal contents outside the abdomen. An inguinal hernia first appears in the lower abdomen at the hip joint area. As it enlarges, it projects into the scrotum. A diaphragmatic hernia is the protrusion of the abdominal contents through the diaphragm into the chest cavity.

SIGNS AND SYMPTOMS

- Diaphragmatic hernia:
  A. Severe type—Bochdalek form—
    - Severe forms appear at birth as respiratory distress.
    - Cyanosis
    - Tachypnea
    - Poorly developed lung
    - Sunken abdomen
  B. Less severe type—Morgagni
    - May have no symptoms
    - Vomiting
    - Chest pain
    - Cough
    - Shortness of breath
- Inguinal hernia:
  - ▶ Swelling in the groin, scrotum, labia that increases with coughing, crying, and urination
  - ▶ Vomiting
  - ▶ Abdominal distention
  - ▶ Abdominal pain

CAUSES

- Diaphragmatic hernia—abnormal development in first trimester
- Inguinal hernia—increased intra-abdominal pressure or weakness of muscles

SCOPE

- Inguinal hernia is common in males (90%) and premature babies.
- Diaphragmatic hernia affects 1 of 2200 to 5000 live births.

 Diagnosis

QUESTIONS THE DOCTOR MAY ASK

- Diaphragmatic hernia:
  Cyanosis—respiratory distress?
  Difficulty breathing?
  Vomiting?
- Inguinal hernia?
  Lump in groin?

WHAT THE DOCTOR LOOKS FOR

- Diaphragmatic hernia:
  Bowel sounds in chest
- Inguinal hernia:
  Mass in groin
  Swelling in scrotum
  Water in scrotum (hydrocele)

TESTS AND PROCEDURES

- Arterial blood tests
- Chest X-ray
- Fetal ultrasound

Treatment

GENERAL MEASURES

Surgical repair is the definitive treatment.

ACTIVITY

N/A

DIET

N/A

 ## Follow-Up

WHAT TO EXPECT

- In most cases, recovery from repair of inguinal hernia is very good.
- Recovery from diaphragmatic hernia depends on the degree of lung damage.

SIGNS TO WATCH

Recurrence of inguinal hernia, appearance on opposite side

PREVENTION

N/A

 ## Common Questions and Answers

Q: Is surgery of great urgency in childhood?
A: Incarceration (obstructed and irreducible) is common in infants less than 1 year, and surgery is recommended early. An irreducible hernia requires urgent surgery. A patient in neonatal intensive care who is receiving continual surveillance for irreducibility can have surgery postponed until the week of discharge or when the neonate can tolerate surgery.

Q: Should bilateral inguinal hernias be repaired at the same time?
A: It depends on the surgeon. There is no evidence that routine exploration of the opposite site reduces the rate of infertility.

Q: What about inguinal hernias in girls?
A: It only occurs in 10% of all inguinal hernias. The overy is the organ commonly found to herniate, and detection is often more difficult. It is often mistaken for adenopathy or lymphadenitis. The ovary can undergo torsion and infarction; 1% of these patients are phenotypic females and have undergone testicular feminization, without an absence of uterus but have a normal XX karyotype.

Herpes

 ## Basics

DESCRIPTION

Herpes simplex virus (HSV) produces a wide spectrum of illness ranging from fever blisters to fatal viral encephalitis.

SIGNS AND SYMPTOMS

- Neonatal infection: Usually acquired from the maternal genitourinary tract during birth and causes serious disease with a high mortality rate. A blistered rash is present at birth or within a few days in almost all infants. Infection may affect the liver, lungs, adrenal glands, and sometimes the central nervous system (CNS). Commonly affects the skin, eyes, or mouth.
- Stomatitis: The most common form of HSV primary infection in children. Fever and irritability precede the development of blister lesions on the lips, gums, and tongue. Children refuse to drink because of the mouth pain and are at risk of dehydration. The child usually starts to improve in 3 to 5 days and recovers in 14 days. Illness may recur.
- Vulvovaginitis: Characterized by fever, headache, malaise, and muscle ache. Local genital symptoms include severe pain, itching, painful urination, and vaginal or urethral discharge. The genital lesions begin as vesicles and progress to ulcers before they crust over. Lesions last for 2 to 3 weeks. Episode may recur.

CAUSE

Infection by herpes virus
- HSV-1: typically lesions of head, neck, and torso
- HSV-2: genital

Each virus can appear in both areas.
- Neonatal herpes: usually type 2

SCOPE

- Herpes infection is widespread; up to 20% of adults may be contagious.
- From 30% to 100% of population subgroups have been exposed to HSV.

 ## Diagnosis

QUESTIONS THE DOCTOR MAY ASK

- Onset of lesions?
- Pain?
- Fever?
- Exposure?
- Fluid intake?
- Encephalitis
  - fever
  - headache
  - seizure
- vaginitis
  - fever
  - pain
  - itching
  - discharge
  - tenderness

WHAT THE DOCTOR LOOKS FOR

The location and type of lesions

TESTS AND PROCEDURES

Viral isolation

Treatment

GENERAL MEASURES

- Antiviral therapy for neonatal infection, vulvovaginitis, and stomatitis
- Acyclovir for encephalitis and vaginitis
- Gingivostomatitis: Most patients are managed with symptomatic therapy, including antifever medication and oral fluids like popsicles. Oral anesthetics can be harmful and result in self-injury when children chew on anesthetized lips.

ACTIVITY

N/A

DIET

N/A

 ## Medications

COMMONLY PRESCRIBED DRUGS

Acyclovir

 ## Follow-Up

WHAT TO EXPECT

- Neonatal infection
  - ▶ The overall mortality rate from untreated neonatal HSV infection is 50%; only 26% of survivors are normal.
  - ▶ The major consequences in survivors are brain damage, seizures, and blindness.
- Stomatitis:
  - ▶ Prognosis is excellent
  - ▶ Acute phase is self-limiting, lasting 4–9 days.
  - ▶ Pain disappears 2–4 days before complete healing of ulcers.

SIGNS TO WATCH

Recurrence of fever, lethargy, dehydration (decreased urine output), worsening of pain, swelling.

PREVENTION

- Neonatal infection: Cesarean section in a mother with active genital herpes at the time of delivery is the main way to prevent neonatal infection.
- Infection after birth:
  - ▶ Adults with oral herpes must be particularly careful to use appropriate hygiene.
  - ▶ Patients with genital lesions from HSV should not have intercourse until the lesions heal.
  - ▶ Condoms can help prevent the spread of HSV but are not completely effective.

 ## Common Questions and Answers

Q: What steps should be taken in the nursery for an infant born to an HSV-positive mother?
A: Neonates with documented perinatal exposure to HSV may be in the incubation phase of infection and should be observed carefully. Infants of mothers with active HSV should be isolated for more than 4–6 hours if they have been delivered vaginally or by cesarean section after membranes were ruptured. The risk of HSV infection in possibly exposed infants (e.g., those born to a mother with a history of recurrent genital herpes) is low, and isolation is not necessary.

Hiccups

 ## Basics

DESCRIPTION

A hiccup is a primitive reflex with no known function. It is an intermittent, involuntary spasm of the diaphragm and chest muscles that results in sudden inspiration, which is abruptly stopped by closure of the glottis.

SIGNS AND SYMPTOMS

- Bout of hiccups: more than a few hiccups, lasting up to 48 hours
- Persistent hiccups: those lasting more than 48 hours
- Intractable hiccups: those lasting more than 1 month

CAUSES

Definitive cause rarely found in infants and children

SCOPE

- Affects all ages
- Third trimester fetus often hiccups.
- More common in the evening
- No known racial, geographic, or socioeconomic variation

 ## Diagnosis

QUESTIONS THE DOCTOR MAY ASK

- Medications, alcohol, and illicit drug use?
- Persistence during sleep?
- Emotional status?

WHAT THE DOCTOR LOOKS FOR

- Physical examination
- Thorough neurologic examination
- Mental status examination

TESTS AND PROCEDURES

None usually indicated; testing indicated if serious associated disease present

 ## Treatment

GENERAL MEASURES

- Treatment is necessary in persistent or severe cases only.
- Noninvasive medical therapy: behavioral conditioning, hypnosis, and acupuncture
- Home remedies: swallowing granulated sugar or breathing into a paper bag
- "Unproved" home remedies: pulling on the tongue, breath holding, ice water gargles, noxious odors or tastes, drinking from the wrong side of a glass, biting on a lemon, rubbing the back of the neck, and inducing the startle reaction
- Invasive physical and surgical maneuvers performed by health professionals. Include stimulation of throat with catheter and nerve blocks.

ACTIVITY

N/A

DIET

N/A

Medications

COMMONLY PRESCRIBED DRUGS

- Chlorpromazine hydrochloride
- Haloperidol
- Metoclopramide
- Phenytoin
- Valproic acid
- Stimulants: ephedrine, methylphenidate, amphetamine, nikethamide

 Follow-Up

WHAT TO EXPECT

- Hiccups due to identifiable cause usually resolve with treatment of the underlying process.
- The prognosis in children is excellent.

SIGNS TO WATCH

- Dehydration
- Exhaustion
- Chest pain
- Palpitations/lightheadedness

PREVENTION

N/A

 Common Questions and Answers

Q: Is it dangerous for my child to frequently hiccup?
A: No, although a medical evaluation should be considered if the hiccups disrupt sleeping and/or eating.

Q: I'm pregnant and I think I feel my unborn child hiccup frequently. Is that a problem?
A: No. Pregnant women frequently note that their child hiccups often.

Q: Is it safe to try home remedies to stop hiccups?
A: Most often yes. Using good common sense to guide you with what home remedies you are willing to try will keep you and your child out of trouble. Most home remedies, while not too effective, are harmless.

High Blood Pressure

 Basics

DESCRIPTION

High blood pressure, or hypertension, in children is defined as having an average systolic (upper) and/or diastolic (lower) pressures above the 95th percentile for age and gender, based on measurements taken on at least three separate occasions.

SIGNS AND SYMPTOMS

- Headache
- Blurry vision
- Nosebleed
- Chest pain
- Weight loss or gain
- Flushing
- Rash

CAUSES

- Hypertension is either primary (essential) or secondary.
- Secondary causes of high blood pressure include kidney, heart, hormone, or neurologic disorders; drugs; obesity
- Burns
- Traction under 10 years of age, kidney disease and narrowing of arteries are major causes of hypertension.

SCOPE

- Primary hypertension is the most common cause of hypertension in adolescents and adults.
- Various rates of hypertension in children have been reported, from 1.2 to 13%, but less than 1% appear to require medication.
- African-American adults have a greater incidence of hypertension. Differences in children, however, are not seen until after age 12.
- Primary hypertension is more likely to develop in individuals with a strong family history of hypertension.

 Diagnosis

QUESTIONS THE DOCTOR MAY ASK

- Past medical history: umbilical artery line, urinary tract infection
- Medications: corticosteroids, cold preparations, oral contraceptives, illicit drugs
- Family history: hypertension, drug use, hormone disorders
- Trauma: blood vessel malformation fistula, traction
- Review of symptoms: other systemic diseases

WHAT THE DOCTOR LOOKS FOR

- Physical examination
  - Eye examination
  - Heart sounds
  - Unusual sound in abdomen or neck
  - Pulse
  - Thyroid palpation

TESTS AND PROCEDURES

- Urinalysis, urine culture
- Blood tests
- Echocardiogram
- Kidney ultrasound
- Specialized urinary system tests
- Kidney scan
- Kidney biopsy

Treatment

GENERAL MEASURES

- Mild primary hypertension may be managed with nonpharmacologic treatment: weight reduction, exercise, sodium restriction, avoidance of certain medications
- Drug therapy should be directed to the cause of secondary hypertension when known.
- Medications may be needed in children with mild-to-moderate hypertension if nonpharmacologic therapy has failed or if severe disease is present.
- Surgery may be recommended.
- Dialysis may be necessary for kidney failure.

ACTIVITY

Exercise is helpful.

DIET

Low-salt diet.

 ## Medications

COMMONLY PRESCRIBED DRUGS

Classes of antihypertensive agents include alpha and beta blockers, diuretics, vasodilators, calcium channel blockers, and angiotensin-converting enzyme (ACE) inhibitors.

 ## Follow-Up

WHAT TO EXPECT

- The reduction of blood pressure with medication should be gradual to avoid side effects.
- The medications cause adverse effects.

SIGNS TO WATCH

Headache, visual problems, irregular heart beat

PREVENTION

N/A

 ## Common Questions and Answers

Q: How does licorice cause hypertension?
A: British licorice contains glycyrrhizinic acid, a substance that causes sodium retention, potassium wasting, and high blood pressure. This substance is not found in most commercially available licorice in the United States.

Q: What percentage of children have renovascular causes for their hypertension?
A: Studies looking at the etiology of hypertension show from 10 to 24% of children may have a renovascular cause. Children under 5 years old are 4 times more likely to have renal artery stenosis than adolescents.

Q: What are the indications for invasive studies such as arterioragraphy?
A: This decision should be individualized and based on the severity of the hypertension, response to medication, the clinical presentation (e.g., neurofibromatosis), and results of other studies. In general, young children and all children with severe, unexplained hypertension should be completely evaluated.

Q: How does one manage mild elevations in blood pressure (130/90) when found in asymptomatic adolescents during a school physical?
A: This individual should have repeat blood pressure determinations before being labeled as hypertensive. If repeat measurements confirm the presence of mild hypertension, nonpharmacologic approaches should be considered after a complete history, a physical examination, and directed laboratory studies.

Histoplasmosis

 Basics

DESCRIPTION

Histoplasmosis is an infection of the lung caused by the fungus *Histoplasma capsulatum,* an organism found in soil, blackbird and pigeon roosts, chicken houses, caves, attics, and old buildings.

SIGNS AND SYMPTOMS

- Often causes no symptoms
- In children, severity of acute pulmonary histoplasmosis can vary:
  - ▶ Mild disease: 80% of patients affected; symptoms include upper respiratory symptoms, low grade fever, and chest pain; the course of the disease is 1–5 days
  - ▶ Moderate disease: symptoms include high fever, productive cough, chest pain, shortness of breath, and hoarseness; lasts approximately 15 days
  - ▶ Severe disease: symptoms include high fever, night sweats, weight loss, cough, chest pain, shortness of breath, and hoarseness; lasts up to 3 weeks

CAUSES

Inhalation of spores of *H. capsulatum*

SCOPE

- The most common systemic fungal infection in the United States
- Endemic to the Ohio and Mississippi river valleys; 80% of the adults in these regions are skin-test positive.

 Diagnosis

QUESTIONS THE DOCTOR MAY ASK

- Travel?
- Cough?
- Fever?
- Chest pain?
- Rash?

WHAT THE DOCTOR LOOKS FOR

- Most patients are asymptomatic.
- Flulike signs and symptoms common

TESTS AND PROCEDURES

- Cultures of blood, sputum, bone marrow
- Chest X-ray
- Skin test
- Blood test for antibodies

 Treatment

GENERAL MEASURES

- Recovery is usually spontaneous and does not require drug therapy.
- Patients with severe or disseminated disease may require treatment with antifungal agents.

ACTIVITY

N/A

DIET

N/A

Medications

COMMONLY PRESCRIBED DRUGS

- Amphotericin
- Ketoconazole

 Follow-Up

WHAT TO EXPECT

- In mild-to-moderate cases not requiring drug therapy, recovery usually occurs in 1 to 2 weeks.
- In cases requiring therapy, improvement is usually noted within 2 weeks.
- In most cases, prognosis is excellent.
- 90% mortality rate within 3 months in patients with acute disease if untreated

SIGNS TO WATCH

Prognosis is excellent in most cases.

PREVENTION

N/A

 Common Questions and Answers

Q: How can histoplasmosis be prevented?
A: Prevention can only be achieved by controlling the environmental factors in the affected areas; there are no vaccines for the prevention of histoplasmosis.

Q: Do patients with histoplasmosis need to be isolated?
A: No isolation of infected patients is required.

HIV Infection & AIDS

 Basics

DESCRIPTION

The human immunodeficiency virus (HIV) is a retrovirus that infects immune system cells, causing cell death and a decline in immune function. A person infected with HIV may develop opportunistic infections, cancer, and neurologic lesions (acquired immunodeficiency syndrome [AIDS]). HIV appears to have direct effects on the central nervous system, the gastrointestinal tract, and other systems.

SIGNS AND SYMPTOMS

- AIDS is a chronic infection with variable course.
- Acute infection: fever, rash, muscle aches, and malaise; this self-limited syndrome occurs about 6–8 weeks after infection.
- Following infection, there is a variable period of time without symptoms.
- Lymph node enlargement persisting longer than 3 months
- Other diseases:
  - ▶ Constitutional: fever lasting more than 1 month, loss of weight, persistent diarrhea, skin rash, severe chronic fatigue
  - ▶ Neurologic disease: dementia, nerve disorders
  - ▶ AIDS-defining opportunistic infections: *Pneumocystis carinii* pneumonia (PCP), toxoplasmosis, candidiasis, tuberculosis, other infections
  - ▶ Cancers: Kaposi sarcoma, non-Hodgkin lymphoma, other cancers

CAUSES

HIV virus

SCOPE

- Sexual contact: male to female transmission more contagious than female to male; anal receptive sex more likely to transmit than vaginal sex.
- Exposure to infected blood: almost always involves intravenous (IV) exposure to infected blood (via transfusions or sharing needles). In occupational exposure, the risk of transmis-

sion from a needlestick injury contaminated with HIV-infected blood is 1 in 300.
- HIV can be transmitted in breast milk.
- More than 90% of pediatric infections are acquired during pregnancy or birth.
- The risk of an HIV-infected mother giving birth to an infected infant is approximately 25% without treatment.
- Of infants infected during pregnancy or birth, 50% are believed infected in the womb; the rest acquire the infection around the time of birth.

 Diagnosis

QUESTIONS THE DOCTOR MAY ASK

- Parental risk factors (IV drug use, sexually transmitted diseases, high-risk sex, transfusions before 1986)
- Frequent infections
- Failure to thrive
- Recurrent/chronic diarrhea
- Recurrent/chronic enlargement of parotid gland

WHAT THE DOCTOR LOOKS FOR

- Physical examination
- Neurologic evaluation
- Enlarged lymph nodes
- Pneumonia
- Large liver or spleen
- Recurrent thrush

TESTS AND PROCEDURES

- Blood tests
- HIV culture and/or polymerase chain reaction (PCR) DNA testing
- Computed tomography (CT), magnetic resonance imaging (MRI)

Treatment

GENERAL MEASURES

- Immunizations
- Antiretroviral therapy
- Immune enhancement
- Prevention of infection
- Psychosocial support for the family is critical. For many families, HIV infection is added to other stressors related to urban life (inadequate finances, hard-to-access health care, inadequate housing and child care, domestic violence, and substance abuse).

ACTIVITY

N/A

DIET

N/A

 ## Medications

COMMONLY PRESCRIBED DRUGS

- Antiretroviral drugs (AZT)
- Antibiotics
- Gamma globulin
- Protease inhibitors
- Trimethoprim/sulfa

 ## Follow-Up

WHAT TO EXPECT

- 25% of infants infected during pregnancy or birth develop early symptomatic disease, with an AIDS diagnosis by 1 to 2 years of life. These children frequently die by 3 years of age.
- The remaining 75% have late onset of symptoms, usually after 5 years of age, and the median survival of this group is now 8–12 years old.

SIGNS TO WATCH

N/A

PREVENTION

- HIV infection is almost completely preventable by avoiding high-risk behaviors.
- It is now possible to significantly decrease the risk to newborns of HIV-infected women. AZT taken by the mother during pregnancy can decreases the risk of transmission of HIV to the fetus. Avoiding breast-feeding is another way to decrease the risk of transmission.

 ## Common Questions and Answers

Q: Once the HIV-exposed infant achieves negative antibody status, how sure are we that he/she is uninfected?
A: With today's technology, if the child has also been PCR and/or blood-culture negative at least twice, and is clinically well, the chance that the child still harbors HIV is very low and appears to be less than 1 per 1000. The child should continue to be followed by a health care provider aware of his/her past HIV antibody status. If conditions warrant, retesting would be an option at a later date.

Hydrocephalus

 Basics

DESCRIPTION

Hydrocephalus is a condition marked by the increased size of ventricles within the brain. It may lead to blindness, nerve dysfunction, signs of increased intracranial pressure, or cognitive impairment. Sometimes called "water on brain."

SIGNS AND SYMPTOMS

- Children may present with headache, lethargy, and vomiting.
- Infants may present with vomiting, lethargy, irritability, rapid increase in head size, and a bulging soft spot (fontanelle).
- Large head
- Loss of color and peripheral vision
- Abnormal pupils and eye movement
- Muscle spasm

CAUSES

- Overproduction of cerebral spinal fluid or blockage of drainage of fluid.
- Birth defect
- Degenerative condition
- Meningitis
- Brain tumors
- Trauma
- Vascular conditions

SCOPE

N/A

 Diagnosis

QUESTIONS THE DOCTOR MAY ASK

- Headache?
- Visual problem?
- Irritability?
- Lethargy?
- Vomiting?
- Record of head size measurements?

WHAT THE DOCTOR LOOKS FOR

- Head size measurements
- Muscle tone
- Reflexes

TESTS AND PROCEDURES

- Magnetic resonance imaging (MRI) of the brain
- Ultrasound of the head
- Serial measurement of head circumference

 Treatment

GENERAL MEASURES

- Surgery
- Shunting of cerebrospinal fluid is frequently necessary when hydrocephalus is progressive or causes symptoms.
- Serial spinal taps may be an alternative to a shunt.

ACTIVITY

N/A

DIET

N/A

Medications

COMMONLY PRESCRIBED DRUGS

Acetazolamide

 Follow-Up

WHAT TO EXPECT

Disabilities vary and depend on the cause of hydrocephalus.

SIGNS TO WATCH

Headache, irritability, lethargy, enlarged head size

PREVENTION

N/A

 Common Questions and Answers

Q: What is evidence of malfunctioning shunt?
A: Irritability, vomiting, personality change, lethargy.

Hydronephrosis

 Basics

DESCRIPTION

Hydronephrosis is an enlargement of the upper urinary tract, the kidney.

SIGNS AND SYMPTOMS

- Abdominal, flank, or back pain
- Blood in urine
- Upper urinary tract infection
- Poor urinary stream or dribbling
- High blood pressure
- Failure to thrive
- Hypertension

CAUSES

- Urinary system obstruction
- Reflux of urine from bladder back into kidney
- Other congenital anomalies

SCOPE

The incidence of congenital hydronephrosis is 0.17–0.93%.

 Diagnosis

QUESTIONS THE DOCTOR MAY ASK

- Fever
- Abdominal pain
- Blood in urine

WHAT THE DOCTOR LOOKS FOR

- Abdominal mass
- Poor urinary stream

TESTS AND PROCEDURES

- Blood tests
- Ultrasound
- Voiding cystourethrography
- Other specialized imaging procedures

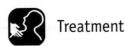

Treatment

GENERAL MEASURES

- Antibiotics
- Surgery to relieve obstruction

ACTIVITY

N/A

DIET

N/A

Medications

COMMONLY PRESCRIBED DRUGS

Antibiotics

Follow-Up

WHAT TO EXPECT

- Urine cultures
- Repeat imaging of renal system
- Blood pressure

SIGNS TO WATCH

Fever, headache, painful urination

PREVENTION

N/A

Common Questions and Answers

Q: How does bleeding occur?
A: The large kidney under presssure will bleed with only minor trauma.

Q: Will surgery completely correct the problem?
A: In some cases it will. In other cases, the dilated renal system does not return to normal size. This situation can still restore good urine output and normal blood tests.

Impetigo

Basics

DESCRIPTION

Impetigo is a superficial infection of the skin that may produce fluid-filled blisters. Impetigo typically begins as a reddened, tender pimple that rapidly progresses into a blister before forming a shallow ulcer covered by a yellowish crust.

SIGNS AND SYMPTOMS

- Begins as a tender red bump or pimple in the skin
- May develop slowly or spread rapidly
- May develop into fluid-filled blisters
- When blisters break, produces weeping, shallow, red ulcer that becomes covered with a honey-colored crust
- Most often occurs on the face around the mouth and nose, or at site of trauma
- May form "satellite lesions" at multiple areas of the body

CAUSES

- Bacterial infection
- May be transmitted by direct contact or by insect bite
- May be result of contamination at site of trauma
- Staph and strep common.

SCOPE

- Most common in warm, humid seasons
- Associated with socioeconomic disadvantage, especially crowding
- Most common bacterial skin infection in children
- Rare under 2 years of age; most common between 2 to 7 years of age; seen in older groups more often as part of an epidemic

Diagnosis

QUESTIONS THE DOCTOR MAY ASK

- Recent trauma (may be minor)?
- Factors that provide permissive environment: warm temperature, high humidity, prior antibiotic use (altering normal skin flora)?
- Altered host immunity?

WHAT THE DOCTOR LOOKS FOR

- Characteristic skin lesions

TESTS AND PROCEDURES

- Culture for microbiologic analysis
- Blood tests and blood culture
- Skin biopsy indicated if diagnosis in question

Treatment

GENERAL MEASURES

- Supportive care
- Cleansing and debriding lesions are not necessary.
- Underlying (predisposing) skin diseases and infestations are treated.
- Spread through a household is common, with children frequently reinfecting themselves and other family members.
- Children with underlying skin disease (e.g., eczema) are difficult to treat because of heavy bacterial skin colonization and trauma to skin from scratching.

ACTIVITY

Avoid engaging in team sports until symptoms resolve.

DIET

N/A

Medications

COMMONLY PRESCRIBED DRUGS

Antibiotics: muciprocin (Bactroban), erythromycin, cefadroxil, dicloxacillin, amoxicillin/clavulanic acid, clindamycin, clarithromycin

 ## Follow-Up

WHAT TO EXPECT

- Nonblistered: If untreated, lesions develop slowly over several weeks and then heal spontaneously; occasionally, ulcers form even when properly treated.
- Blistered: Blisters usually rupture spontaneously and then heal over a period of several days to 1 week when properly treated.

SIGNS TO WATCH

- Development of deeper infection
- Fever
- Persistence or recurrence of impetigo

PREVENTION

- Impetigo is very contagious and often spreads through households and athletic teams.
- Hand washing is very important.
- Cut fingernails to prevent scratching; use gloves at night.
- Give child separate sleeping quarters and clothing until lesions resolved.

 ## Common Questions and Answers

Q: What should be done with a child who continues to have impetigo despite repeated courses of antibiotics?
A: A search for a household source who is reinfecting the patient is probably most important. Underlying skin diseases should be treated if possible, and other diagnoses suspected if there is no improvement.

Q: Should the child be isolated from other family members and kept from school?
A: Until the lesions are treated, close contact of the child with other people should be discouraged (e.g., separate sleeping quarters, clothing, etc.). The child may return to school but should not participate in activities with close physical contact (sports) until treated.

Immune Thrombocytopenic Purpura

Basics

DESCRIPTION

Immune thrombocytopenic purpura is a deficiency of platelets, a blood component responsible for clotting, due to destruction caused by circulating antiplatelet antibodies. It can lead to bleeding within the brain, eyes, gastrointestinal tract, or other areas of the body.

- Classified as acute when resolving in less than 12 months, otherwise chronic (and/or recurring)
- May occur alone or in association with other autoimmune symptoms

SIGNS AND SYMPTOMS

- Often preceded by a viral infection 1–3 weeks before onset of symptoms
- Bruising and red spots appear suddenly in an otherwise healthy child.
- Increased skin bleeding, nosebleed, blood in urine, gastrointestinal bleeding

CAUSES

- Cause of antibody production is usually unknown.
- Immune response (virus or drugs) may produce antibodies that cross-react with platelets.

SCOPE

- Most common acquired platelet disorder of childhood
- Incidence is approximately 30 per 1,000,000 children under 15 years of age
- Slight seasonal peaks in winter and spring

Diagnosis

QUESTIONS THE DOCTOR MAY ASK

- Drugs which lower platelets, aspirin, heparin seizure medication
- Severity of bleeding
- Dark stools or red urine
- Risk factors for HIV
- Neurologic problems

WHAT THE DOCTOR LOOKS FOR

- The degree of production and destruction of platelets
- Signs and symptoms of chronic disease
- Other autoimmune diseases
- Neurologic exam
- Abdominal exam
- Effect of bleeding in brain
- Spleen enlargement

TESTS AND PROCEDURES

- Blood tests
- Sample of bone marrow
- Special blood-clotting studies

Treatment

GENERAL MEASURES

- Therapy is aimed at preventing serious bleeding during the period of thrombocytopenia, which is generally self-limited.
- Avoidance of antiplatelet medications (aspirin, ibuprofen, cold medications with antihistamines)
- Observation alone is safe for most older children without serious bleeding, who have reliable caretakers, and in whom adequate supervision and follow-up are assured.
- Filtration of the blood (plasmapheresis) may be recommended.
- In certain circumstances (active toddlers, persistent bleeding) medications may be necessary.
- Surgery: not indicated for ITP. In chronic TP when spleens are removed, 70–80% of patients respond to removal of the spleen, but there are no predictors of response before surgery.
- Life-threatening bleeding requires emergency management.

ACTIVITY

Age-appropriate precautions to prevent trauma (e.g., limited activity, helmet use) should be instituted.

DIET

N/A

Medications

COMMONLY PRESCRIBED DRUGS

- Corticosteroids
- Intravenous immunoglobulin (IVIG)
- Anti-D immunoglobulin
- Other immune system suppression agents: azathioprine, cyclophosphamide, cyclosporine, vincristine, danazol, monoclonal anti-Fc receptor

Follow-Up

WHAT TO EXPECT

- Spontaneous recovery is the norm (60% by 3 months, 75% by 6 months, and approximately 90% by 1 year).
- The incidence of significant bleeding-related complications and mortality is extremely low.
- Of patients with chronic disease, approximately 20% ultimately have spontaneous resolution of their thrombocytopenia, even as long as 10–20 years after diagnosis. Bleeding-related mortality rate is under 5%.

SIGNS TO WATCH

Parents should be educated about the signs and symptoms of increased intracranial pressure.

Common Questions and Answers

Q: Why aren't platelet transfusions used to increase the platelet count?
A: Because antiplatelet antibodies continue to be produced in patients with immune thrombocytopenic purpura, transfused platelets are rapidly consumed and no increase in platelet counts is observed.

Q: Will the thrombocytopenic purpura recur after another viral infection?
A: In a minority of patients, recurrence follows a subsequent viral infection, but most patients continue to maintain normal platelet counts once their illness has resolved.

Q: Should *all* activities be limited until the platelet count returns to normal?
A: A common sense approach to activities should prevail. It is clear that bleeding within the brain can occur even in the absence of any trauma, so unreasonable restrictions are not advised. One rule of thumb for children with low platelet counts is to avoid any activity where one foot is not on the ground at all times.

Infantile Spasms

 Basics

DESCRIPTION

Infantile spasms are seizures, usually occurring in clusters.

SIGNS AND SYMPTOMS

- Loss of consciousness
- Uncontrollable contraction of muscle
- Incontinence

CAUSES

- Neurologic disorders
- Down syndrome
- Metabolic disorders (congenital lactic acidoses, phenylketonuria [PKU])
- Almost any cause of prenatal or perinatal brain injury may lead to infantile spasms.
- Tuberous sclerosis

SCOPE

- Infantile spasms affect 0.25–0.42 per 1000 live births.
- Peak age of onset is 4–9 months; onset usually occurs before 1 year of age.
- Boys are more often affected than girls.

 Diagnosis

QUESTIONS THE DOCTOR MAY ASK

- Prenatal and perinatal history
- Family history
- Developmental history
- Physical examination
- Neurologic evaluation

WHAT THE DOCTOR LOOKS FOR

- Down syndrome
- Large liver/spleen
- Skin lesions
- Mental status

TESTS AND PROCEDURES

- Electroencephalogram (EEG)
- Blood tests
- If no cause is found, lumbar puncture (spinal tap)
- Magnetic resonance imaging (MRI), computed tomography (CT)
- Cardiologic evaluation
- Kidney ultrasound
- Genetic evaluation

 Treatment

GENERAL MEASURES

N/A

ACTIVITY

N/A

DIET

N/A

Medications

COMMONLY PRESCRIBED DRUGS

- Adrenocorticotropic hormone (ACTH)
- Antiseizure drugs: clonazepam, phenobarbital, valproate
- Prednisone
- Pyridoxine

 Follow-Up

WHAT TO EXPECT

- Infantile spasms carry a poor developmental prognosis.
- Approximately 65–90% of patients are developmentally delayed at the time of initial diagnosis, and perhaps 10% of these children achieve normal cognitive, physical, and educational development.
- Approximately 55–65% of children with infantile spasms go on to develop other seizure types.
- Of those with an unknown cause, up to 40% having normal cognitive development and freedom from seizures on long-term follow-up.

SIGNS TO WATCH

N/A

PREVENTION

N/A

 Common Questions and Answers

Q: Do infantile spasms ever remit spontaneously?
A: Spontaneous remission of infantile spasms has been reported but appears to be rare.

Q: What predictions can be made about the prognosis of the child with idiopathic (unknown cause) infantile spasms?
A: Periodic evaluation by a child neurologist or child developmentalist helps to detect delays in motor or cognitive development; neither the EEG nor any other laboratory test contributes predictive information in infantile spasms of unknown cause.

Inflammatory Bowel Disease

 Basics

DESCRIPTION

Inflammatory bowel disease, also called Crohn disease, is a chronic inflammatory disease that can affect the entire gastrointestinal tract. It can lead to obstruction, infection, failure to thrive, and other serious complications.

SIGNS AND SYMPTOMS

- Weight loss
- Diarrhea
- Abdominal pain
- Rectal bleeding
- Growth failure
- Nausea and vomiting
- Rectal disease
- Arthritis, mouth ulcers, kidney stones, blood-clotting disorders, other conditions

CAUSES

Unknown

SCOPE

- Average age of onset of Crohn disease in children is 7.5 years (5.9 years in ulcerative colitis).
- Incidence rate is 3.5 per 100,000 North American 10–19 year olds.
- 20–25% patients first present in childhood or adolescence.
- Males and females are equally affected.
- Having a first-degree relative with the illness carries a 5–25% higher risk.
- Family members of patients with Crohn disease have increased risk for both Crohn disease and ulcerative colitis.
- Concordance in monozygotic twins is high.

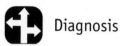 Diagnosis

QUESTIONS THE DOCTOR MAY ASK

- Diarrhea
- Abdominal pain
- Weight loss
- Rectal bleeding
- Growth measurements
- Mouth sores

WHAT THE DOCTOR LOOKS FOR

Symptoms depend on the site of disease activity.

TESTS AND PROCEDURES

- Blood tests
- Stool analysis
- Urinalysis
- X-ray of abdomen
- Upper gastrointestinal (GI) series
- Computed tomography (CT) and ultrasound
- Endoscopy

Treatment

GENERAL MEASURES

- Bowel rest with intravenous (parenteral) nutrition
- Elemental diet has reported to be effective in inducing remission in active disease. Because of its unpalatableness and lack of clear efficacy, its use to induce remission in children is not universally recommended.
- To correct growth failure, an increase in caloric intake of 40% is recommended and can be given as overnight nasogastric feedings if oral supplements are not tolerated. An elemental formula is recommended.
- Drug therapy
- Surgery may be considered.

 ## Medications

COMMONLY PRESCRIBED DRUGS

- Prednisone
- Sulfasalazine
- Asacol
- Pentasa
- Dipentum
- Rowasa
- Metronidazole
- Azathioprine
- Cyclosporine
- Topical hydrocortisone (liquid and foam enemas)

 ## Follow-Up

WHAT TO EXPECT

- This disease is associated with a high degree of illness.
- The majority of patients experience recurring disease.
- In adults, 55% of patients have mild-to-severe disease at any one time with the remainder in remission.
- Patients with colonic disease seem to suffer more from other diseases and are more resistant to treatment.
- Disease may be worsened by viral illness.
- Death is a rare complication.
- After 5 and 20 years of disease, the probability of survival is 98 and 89% of expected survival, respectively.

SIGNS TO WATCH

- Weight loss
- Abdominal pain
- Rectal bleeding

PREVENTION

N/A

 ## Common Questions and Answers

Q: What problems outside of the intestine may occur?
A: Arthritis, deep skin sores, mouth ulcers, eye pain, kidney stones.

Q: What causes poor weight gain?
A: Poor appetite, malabsorbtion, increased energy expenditure and prolonged corticosteroid use.

Iron Deficiency Anemia

 Basics

DESCRIPTION

Decrease in hemoglobin production from decreased iron intake or excessive losses of blood. Other forms of anemia are related to the poor absorption or utilization of iron. The onset of iron deficiency anemia may be acute with rapid blood loss, or chronic with poor diet or slow blood loss. Iron deficiency anemia is the most common cause of anemia in the United States.

SIGNS AND SYMPTOMS

- Iron deficiency anemia initially causes no symptoms.
- Dry, peeling lips
- Shortness of breath
- Fatigue, listlessness
- Rapid heart rate, palpitations
- Pallor
- Blue sclera (whites of eyes)
- Headache
- Irritability, inability to concentrate
- Pain or tingling sensation in extremities
- Susceptibility to infection

CAUSES

- Blood loss (e.g., menstruation, gastrointestinal bleeding)
- Poor iron intake
- Poor iron absorption
- Increased demand for iron (e.g., infancy, adolescence)
- Hookworms

SCOPE

- Variable depending on the groups studied and definition used.
- Prevalence generally between 1 and 8%.
- Most common cause of anemia, predominantly in ages at which there is rapid growth (e.g., infancy, adolescence), and especially in adolescent girls

 Diagnosis

QUESTIONS THE DOCTOR MAY ASK

- How much cow's milk does the child drink per day?
- Diet, especially iron—rich food like oily fish, meat, and iron-containing formula?
- Prematurity?
- Early introduction of cow's milk into diet of infant?
- Gastrointestinal blood loss, nose bleeds?

WHAT THE DOCTOR LOOKS FOR

- The presence and degree of anemia
- Physical examination: paleness, rapid heart rate, GI blood loss

TESTS AND PROCEDURES

- Blood tests
- Bone marrow sample
- Hemoccult tests for blood in stool may be done at home.

 Treatment

GENERAL MEASURES

- Diet
- May require initial inpatient observation in cases of severe anemia
- Blood transfusion is rarely necessary.

ACTIVITY

N/A

DIET

- Educate family regarding age-appropriate diet, including adequate iron.
- Foods high in ascorbic acid increase iron absorption (e.g., orange juice).
- Infants should receive iron-containing formula until 1 year of age.
- Breast-fed infants: For full-term infants, iron supplementation is not recommended until 6 months of age if breast-feeding continues beyond that time.

Medications

COMMONLY PRESCRIBED DRUGS

Ferrous sulfate

 Follow-Up

WHAT TO EXPECT

- Patients should show recovery of a normal hemoglobin and iron stores with adequate oral replacement therapy.
- Long-term prognosis is a function of subsequent diet.
- Some evidence suggests that some of the cognitive dysfunction suffered by patients with iron deficiency may be long-lasting.
- Blood tests should be repeated at 1 month after treatment.

SIGNS TO WATCH

- Shock: cardiovascular failure in cases of severe anemia (rare)
- Psychomotor development and cognitive function

PREVENTION

N/A

Common Questions and Answers

Q: My child will only drink milk. What can I do?
A: Often children do not eat their meals because they have "filled up" on milk or juice before the meal. One option is to not offer any liquids until after the child has eaten a meal. A good general rule of thumb, however, is to never make meal time a battle. Always offer the child a variety of healthful foods from which to choose. Then let the child pick the foods he/she wants to eat. Do not insist that the child "clean his/her plate." Consider allowing the child to make some of the meal choices him/herself. Most of all, do not get discouraged if the child initially refuses to eat. Just hang in there and *be consistent.*

Q: Will the iron medicine stain my child's teeth?
A: The liquid preparation may temporarily stain teeth. Staining is less likely to occur if the medicine is diluted.

Q: Why does my child have to take the iron for 4 to 5 months?
A: It takes this long to fully replenish all the iron stores in the body.

Q: Should the child take vitamins? Vitamins with iron?
A: Different pediatricians have differing views on the relative need of daily vitamins. While the child is taking therapeutic iron, there is no need for supplemental vitamins with iron. After the iron therapy is completed, a daily over-the-counter vitamin with iron certainly won't hurt, but the more important emphasis should be placed on giving the child and teaching the child to eat healthful meals with plenty of fruits and vegetables. A child who is eating this type of diet does not need supplemental vitamins.

Irritable Bowel Syndrome

 Basics

DESCRIPTION

Irritable bowel syndrome (IBS), also called spastic or irritable colon, is a set of signs and symptoms of altered bowel habits, abdominal pain, and gaseousness in the absence of other disease.

SIGNS AND SYMPTOMS

- Most patients have all signs and symptoms, but not with every episode.
- Abdominal pain, usually lower quadrant, relieved by defecation
- Mucus in stools
- Constipation
- Diarrhea
- Distention
- Upper abdominal discomfort after eating
- Straining for normal consistency stools
- Urgency of defecation
- Feeling of incomplete evacuation
- Hard, round stool
- Nausea, vomiting (rare)

CAUSES

The cause of IBS is unknown.

SCOPE

- IBS is thought to occur in 15–30% of the general population.
- 50% of patients present with symptoms before age 35, and 33% can trace their symptoms back into childhood.
- More common in females

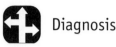 Diagnosis

QUESTIONS THE DOCTOR MAY ASK

- Factors that make symptoms better or worse?
- A detailed diet and travel history?
- The severity and quality of abdominal pain and distention?

WHAT THE DOCTOR LOOKS FOR

- A change in their bowel habits, at times leading to bouts of alternating diarrhea and constipation.
- Often, individuals with IBS can identify certain events that exacerbate or trigger an episode. These triggers may include stress, anxiety, certain foods (wheats, milk, alcohol, caffeine), and cigarette smoking.
- Physical examination

TESTS AND PROCEDURES

- Blood tests
- Urinalysis
- Abdominal X-ray
- Endoscopy and colonoscopy

Treatment

GENERAL MEASURES

- The best treatment for IBS is reassurance of both the parents and the child.
- The symptoms are not dangerous to the child.
- Psychotherapy may be tried. In this therapy, patients are taught a variety of techniques and exercises to use during the episodes of pain that allow them to focus on other subjects and not focus on the pain.
- Eliminating factors that trigger episodes can reduce or eliminate symptoms.

ACTIVITY

N/A

DIET

Fiber supplementation

 ## Medications

COMMONLY PRESCRIBED DRUGS

- Dicyclomine (Bentyl)
- Hyoscyamine (Levsin)
- Donnetal
- Mebeverine
- Amitriptyline
- Imodium
- Lorazepam

 ## Follow-Up

WHAT TO EXPECT

There is no standard or specific follow-up needed for those with IBS.

SIGNS TO WATCH

N/A

PREVENTION

N/A

 ## Common Questions and Answers

Q: Is there a genetic inheritance with IBS?
A: Although family inheritance patterns exist, no specific data are available.

Q: Are there any personality traits identified that are more likely to develop IBS?
A: Adult studies suggest a predilection for certain types; no studies in children.

Kawasaki Disease

 Basics

DESCRIPTION

Kawasaki disease is a multisystem disease of unknown cause affecting young children, characterized by inflammation of small- and medium-sized blood vessels. It can lead to the development of an aneurysm, a thinning and ballooning of a blood vessel.

SIGNS AND SYMPTOMS

- Fever for more than 5 days
- Reddened eyes (pink eye)
- Rash
- Upper respiratory tract: swelling and fissures of the lips, crusting of the lips and mouth, a strawberry tongue
- Swelling and reddening of the hands and feet
- Swollen lymph nodes in neck, often only on one side

CAUSES

- Cause is uncertain.
- The clinical and epidemiologic profile of the disease suggests an infectious agent.
- Association with recent use of rug cleaners or having had rugs shampooed has not been substantiated.

SCOPE

- Average age of cases is 2.3 years with 80% of cases in children less than 4 years of age. 5% of cases occur in children greater than 10 years of age; almost unheard of in children over age 15.
- Recurrence is low (approximately 0.8%).
- In the United States, incidence seems to be increasing (approximately 11% per year in the period 1984–1990).

 Diagnosis

QUESTIONS THE DOCTOR MAY ASK

- Onset of fever?
- Type of rash?
- Diarrhea?
- Joint pain?

WHAT THE DOCTOR LOOKS FOR

- Recognizable phases of typical presentation
- The presence of aneurysms
- Physical examination
- Lymph node enlargement
- Mouth lesions
- Rash
- Swollen joints
- Swelling of legs

TESTS AND PROCEDURES

- Slit lamp eye examination
- Blood tests
- Urinalysis
- Lumbar puncture (spinal tap)
- Electrocardiogram (EKG)
- Chest X-ray
- Echocardiogram

 Treatment

GENERAL MEASURES

- Blood tests should be done every week or two until they return to normal.
- In patients with aneurysms, EKG, chest X-ray, echocardiogram, and other heart function tests should be done at regular intervals.

ACTIVITY

Children with Kawasaki disease should be kept on bedrest until the second or third week of illness or when they have been afebrile for over 72 hours. Bedrest is necessary due to the possibility of myocardial involvement during the acute phase.

DIET

N/A

Medications

COMMONLY PRESCRIBED DRUGS

- Intravenous immunoglobulin (IVIG)
- Aspirin
- Dipyridamole

Follow-Up

WHAT TO EXPECT

- The natural course of Kawasaki disease is a gradual improvement.
- With IVIG, children usually show marked resolution of clinical symptoms within 2 to 3 days of treatment (70–80%).
- Without treatment with IVIG, 15–25% of patients develop coronary aneurysms.
- Death occurs secondary to cardiac disease in 0.3–2% of cases.
- Myocardial infarction can occur several years after the initial illness.
- Patients who are young (less than 1 year of age), male, and whose fevers persist for greater than 14 days are more likely to develop aneurysms.

SIGNS TO WATCH

Symptoms of cardiac insufficiency (fatigue, chest pain, shortness of breath on exertion)

PREVENTION

- Because the exact cause of Kawasaki disease is unknown, there are no preventive measures that can be employed.
- Isolation of patients is not indicated.

Common Questions and Answers

Q: Do coronary artery aneurysms associated with Kawasaki disease ever resolve?
A: Most coronary artery aneurysms do resolve. Even some giant aneurysms (those greater than 8 millimeters in diameter) will resolve; there is concern, however, that even if aneurysms resolve, these patients may be at risk for the early development of hardening of the arteries (atherosclerosis).

Lactose Intolerance

 Basics

DESCRIPTION

Lactose intolerance is the inability to digest lactose sugar because of the deficiency of the enzyme lactase, resulting in gastrointestinal symptoms. Lactose is a sugar found commonly in dairy products.

SIGNS AND SYMPTOMS

Classic symptoms include bloating, gaseousness, colicky abdominal pain, and diarrhea.

CAUSE

Deficiency of lactose enzyme. May have temporary episode after first diarrhea.

SCOPE

- Deficiency is found in up to 80% of native Australians, Americans, tropical Africans, and East and Southeastern Asians. It is also highly prevalent in African-Americans.
- Seen in cystic fibrosis and protein intolerance.

 Diagnosis

QUESTIONS THE DOCTOR MAY ASK

- Bloating?
- Gaseousness?
- Abdominal pain?
- Diarrhea?
- A detailed diet history?

WHAT THE DOCTOR LOOKS FOR

- Symptoms vary in severity and with dose of lactose.
- Association with milk ingestion may not be evident.
- Physical examination
- Height and weight
- Distended abdomen

TESTS AND PROCEDURES

- Stool analysis
- Lactose breath hydrogen test
    - Measurement of hydrogen in breath. Hydrogen is produced by fermented unabsorbed carbohydrate.

Treatment

GENERAL MEASURES

- Removal of lactose from the diet is effective in eliminating symptoms. However, a milk-free diet may result in calcium deficiency and other nutritional issues.
- Predigestion of lactose can be done by the addition of commercially available enzyme supplementation. Many products are available over the counter. Liquid preparations, capsules, and chewable tablets can be obtained.

ACTIVITY

N/A

DIET

Avoid lactose and milk products; use enzyme supplement before eating milk-containing meals.

 ## Medications

COMMONLY PRESCRIBED DRUGS

N/A

WHAT TO EXPECT

- The majority of patients with lactose intolerance do not recover the ability to digest lactose.
- Some acquired deficiencies, particularly those associated with infection, may resolve over time.
- With lactose avoidance or with enzyme supplementation, the child can control and eliminate symptoms.

SIGNS TO WATCH

N/A

PREVENTION

Avoid foods containing lactose.

 ## Common Questions and Answers

Q: What causes falsely positive hydrogen breath tests?
A: Inadequate fasting prior to test, rapid intestinal transit, toothpaste, bacterial overgrowth and smoking.

Q: When my child had diarrhea, he seemed to be worse when he drank milk. Is this lactose intolerance?
A: Quite likely it is transitory lactose intolerance, which is commonly seen in acute viral diarrhea.

Lazy Eye

Basics

DESCRIPTION

Lazy eye, or amblyopia, is a condition unique to infancy and childhood resulting in decreased vision in one or both eyes. It is caused by any condition resulting in abnormal or unequal visual input between birth and about 9 years of age.

SIGNS AND SYMPTOMS

- Visual loss in one or both eyes
- Eyes not pointed in the same direction

CAUSE

Multiple—anatomic, refractional, genetic—accomodation problems.

SCOPE

Amblyopia is present in 2% of the population and is the leading cause of preventable visual loss in children.

Diagnosis

QUESTIONS THE DOCTOR MAY ASK

- How, when, and where was visual loss first noticed?
- How has this changed?
- Other eye abnormalities noted or treated?
- Family eye history?
- The presence of any trauma, medical, or surgical problems?
- Current and past medications and known allergies?
- Exposures to toxins or new climates/travel/day care or recent illness?

WHAT THE DOCTOR LOOKS FOR

- Visual testing with eye charts
- The doctor will evaluate head posture, eye position and movement, pupillary responses, and other reflexes.
- A general developmental and neurologic examination helps rule out other disease.

TESTS AND PROCEDURES

- Visual evoked responses
- Electroretinography
- Visual tests: eye charts

Treatment

GENERAL MEASURES

- Treatment is directed toward reversing or decreasing the visual stimulus, often with glasses or an eye patch.
- Many children do not tolerate a patch, although alternatives are inadequate.
- Eye drops may be prescribed.
- Other medical management or surgery may be recommended.
- The effectiveness of treatment should be monitored closely because the most common reason for a poor response from an eye patch is noncompliance. Frequent visits provide positive reinforcement, reassurance, and encouragement needed by both the family and the patient.
- Surgery

ACTIVITY

N/A

DIET

N/A

 ## Medications

COMMONLY PRESCRIBED DRUGS

- Atropine eye drops
- L-dopa

 ## Follow-Up

WHAT TO EXPECT

- The earlier amblyopia is identified and treated, the more favorable the outcome.
- The compliance rate with eye patch therapy is 50%, effectively reducing the chance for normal vision.

SIGNS TO WATCH

N/A

PREVENTION

Screening children as soon as possible, by testing vision in school and by the primary care physician, is currently the best method of identifying possible amblyopia and improving the outcome.

 ## Common Questions and Answers

Q: What will be the final vision of an amblyopic eye?
A: The greater the visual difference between the two eyes, the less the chance of achieving normal vision.

Q: Will the eye see normal after successful treatment?
A: An amblyopic eye that is 20/20 after treatment remains subjectively different from the normal eye to the patient for his or her lifetime.

Lead Poisoning

Basics

DESCRIPTION

Lead poisoning results from the chronic exposure to lead. Lead poisoning in children is defined by the Centers for Disease Control as a blood lead level of greater than 10 micrograms per deciliter (mg/dL). Lead typically is absorbed through the gastrointestinal system and distributed through the body into the blood, soft tissues, and bone. Lead poisoning can lead to cognitive and behavioral disturbances, among many other complications.

SIGNS AND SYMPTOMS

- Most children with elevated lead levels are completely symptom-free.
- When symptoms occur, they are nonspecific and may be attributed to a viral illness.
- Symptoms can include abdominal pain, constipation, poor appetite, and vomiting.
- Altered mental status and seizures
- Anemia

CAUSES

- Exposure occurs by ingestion of lead-based paint chips or contaminated dust and soil.
- High-risk properties are homes built before 1960 with peeling paint or those undergoing renovation.
- Window sills may contain high levels of dust containing lead, formed by the repeated opening and closing of windows.
- Soil and dust may contain lead from leaded gasoline or industrial exposures. Although lead-containing gasoline has been largely eliminated, the lead deposited in the past in soil and dust does not break down and remains a constant source of exposure.

- Lead is present within the distribution system of drinking water, particularly in copper pipes with lead-soldered joints or cisterns with lead liners that store water.
- Lead in food may occur from lead-soldered cans, ceramic vessels made with lead glazes, and leaded crystal.
- Miscellaneous sources include folk remedies, stained glass, pottery, and furniture refinishing products.

SCOPE

- 17% of children from 6 months to 5 years of age have levels greater than 15 mg/dL.
- Children living in homes built before 1960 (when lead paint was used) where paint is peeling or renovations are occurring are most likely to have elevated lead levels.
- Siblings of playmates of children with elevated lead levels are at increased risk for lead poisoning.
- Elevated lead levels are more common in the summer and fall.

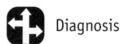

Diagnosis

QUESTIONS THE DOCTOR MAY ASK

- School problems?
- Signs and symptoms of lead poisoning?
- Opportunity for lead exposure in the home or elsewhere?
- Acute onset of vomiting, abnormal mental status, or seizures?
- Exposure to lead of all family members?
- Developmental delay?

WHAT THE DOCTOR LOOKS FOR

- Majority of patients with chronic lead exposure have completely normal physical examinations.
- Mental status changes or other neurologic symptoms

TESTS AND PROCEDURES

- Blood tests
- Urinalysis
- X-ray of abdomen and/or extremities
- Lead level, CBC

Treatment

GENERAL MEASURES

Chelation therapy

ACTIVITY

N/A

DIET

- Children with lead poisoning should receive a diet rich in iron and calcium.
- Many of these children benefit from a daily multivitamin with iron.

Medications

COMMONLY PRESCRIBED DRUGS

- BAL (dimercaprol)
- $CaNa_2$ EDTA
- Chemet (Succimer, DMSA)
- D-Penicillamine

Follow-Up

WHAT TO EXPECT

- In general, children with lead levels between 10 and 20 mg/dL are followed every 3–4 months and counseled to eliminate possible sources of exposure; children with lead levels between 20 and 44 mg/dL should have a full house inspection by the city with lead abatement done by professionals.
- Any child with a lead level greater than 70 mg/dL or with symptoms of lead poisoning must be hospitalized and treated with chelation. The child must not return home until the source of lead is removed.

PREVENTION

- Screening of children is done between the ages of 6 months and 6 years.
- Source of lead must be removed by experts trained in lead removal.
- Minimize lead exposure by wet-mopping floors and cleaning window areas frequently with high-phosphate cleaners.
- Childrens' hands should be washed frequently, especially before eating.
- Toys and pacifiers must be cleaned regularly.
- Water from the tap should be fully flushed before drinking. Because hot water may increase lead absorption, only cold water should be used, even when making formula.

Common Questions and Answers

Q: Is there a "safe" blood lead level?
A: Effects of lead on cognitive functioning can occur at levels as low as 10 mg/dL. It is unclear at present whether blood lead levels of less than 10 mg/dL cause adverse consequences.

Q: When is the recommended period to obtain screening blood lead levels?
A: Children with risk factors for lead (old housing, current renovations, siblings/playmates with high lead, parents in lead-related jobs) should initially be screened at age 6 months until the age of 72 months. Screening should continue past the age of 6 years in children with developmental delays with extensive hand-to-mouth activity or pica.

Leukemia

 Basics

DESCRIPTION

Leukemia is a cancerous proliferation of white blood cells. Acute lymphoblastic leukemia (ALL) is the most common cancer of childhood. Another common form is acute myeloid leukemia (AML).

SIGNS AND SYMPTOMS

- Fever
- Bleeding disorders
- Bone pain
- Fatigue and pallor
- Joint pain, limping
- Purplish skin lesions
- Enlarged gums
- Enlarged lymph nodes
- Symptoms of central nervous system disease: vomiting, headache, seizures
- Shortness of breath
- Scanty urine output

CAUSES

Causes of leukemia are unknown, but may be related to exposure to ionizing radiation, chemicals, viruses, prolonged immune suppression therapy, and other factors.

SCOPE

- Acute lymphoblastic leukemia affects 4 per 100,000 children less than 5 years of age.
- More than 75% of acute childhood leukemia is ALL.
- Peak incidence of ALL is 4 years of age; more common in Caucasians and boys.
- AML accounts for 15 to 20% of childhood acute leukemia.
- Leukemia during first month of life is usually AML.
- Incidence of AML increases in teens.

 Diagnosis

QUESTIONS THE DOCTOR MAY ASK

- Fever?
- Bleeding?
- Bone pain?
- Large lymph nodes?
- Difficulty breathing?

WHAT THE DOCTOR LOOKS FOR

- Large spleen
- Bruises
- Bone pain
- Focus of infection

TESTS AND PROCEDURES

- Blood tests
- Bone marrow sample
- Chest X-ray
- Lumbar puncture (spinal tap)

 Treatment

GENERAL MEASURES

- Chemotherapy
- Supportive care: hydration
- Blood transfusion may be necessary.

ACTIVITY

Keep child undergoing chemotherapy isolated from those with chickenpox or obvious illness.

DIET

N/A

Medications

COMMONLY PRESCRIBED DRUGS

- Chemotherapy agents
- Antibiotics
- Alkalinization agents

 ## Follow-Up

WHAT TO EXPECT

- Maintenance chemotherapy for ALL may last for up to 3 years.
- Remission rate for ALL is 95%.
- Long-term survival rate from ALL is approximately 70%.
- Remission rate for AML is 85% with chemotherapy.
- Approximately 30–40% of patients with AML achieve long-term survival.

SIGNS TO WATCH

Recurrence of symptoms

PREVENTION

N/A

 ## Common Questions and Answers

Q: Are repeated hospitalizations required for children with AML?
A: Repeated hospitalizations are needed for chemotherapy and infections.

Q: Can the child go to school?
A: The child with ALL can go to school while on treatment. The child with AML may attend school intermittently during therapy.

Q: Will the hair fall out and child be sick for all 3 years of chemotherapy for ALL?
A: Hair usually falls out in the first 6 months. Most children feel well during maintenance therapy.

Q: Does the child with ALL need to be isolated from other children?
A: The child should be isolated from any child who has chickenpox or who is obviously sick.

Q: What do we do if we skip a dose of maintenance chemotherapy?
A: Continue to take the medication as recommended. Skipping one dose does not increase risk of relapse. However, missing doses should not become a habit.

Lice

 Basics

DESCRIPTION

Head lice, or pediculosis, is an infestation by parasites that feed on human blood. A mature female louse lays eggs, or nits, which appear as small white spots cemented to the base of hair. Lice may affect head, body, or the pubic hair.

SIGNS AND SYMPTOMS

- Head lice (pediculosis capitis):
  - ▶ Found most often on the back of the head and neck and behind the ears
  - ▶ Nits are white spots on hair shaft that cannot be moved.
  - ▶ Itching
  - ▶ Prickling sensation of the scalp
  - ▶ Eyelashes may be involved.
- Body lice (pediculosis corporis):
  - ▶ Affects individuals with poor hygiene
  - ▶ Adult lice live and lay their nits in the seams of clothing.
  - ▶ Most common symptom is itching that leads to scratching and infection.
  - ▶ Uninfected bites appear as red spots.

- Pubic lice (phthirius pubis) (crabs):
  - ▶ Itching of groin and rectal area
  - ▶ May have no symptoms during 30-day incubation period
  - ▶ Delay in treatment may lead to development of widespread groin inflammation and infection.
  - ▶ Pubic hair most common site
  - ▶ Lice may spread to hair around rectum, abdomen, armpit, chest, beard, eyebrows, and eyelashes.
  - ▶ Infested adult patients may spread lice to eyelashes of children.

CAUSES

Lice are transmitted by close personal contact and contact with objects such as combs, hats, clothing, and bed linen.

SCOPE

- Head lice:
  - ▶ Common in day-care setting and elementary-school children.
  - ▶ Affects all socioeconomic groups
  - ▶ Not indicative of poor hygiene
  - ▶ Slightly higher incidence in girls
- Body lice:
  - ▶ Found on persons with poor hygiene
  - ▶ More common in extreme conditions such as crowding, homelessness, wars, famine, flood, and earthquakes
- Pubic lice:
  - ▶ Most common in adolescents and young adults

 Diagnosis

QUESTIONS THE DOCTOR MAY ASK

- Exposure in school or family?
- Pruritus (itching), which is the hallmark of all lice infestation?
- The presence of lice and/or nits?
- Secondary skin lesion (from scratching)?
- Review of symptoms?

WHAT THE DOCTOR LOOKS FOR

- Up to 50% of individuals with pubic lice have another sexually transmitted disease, particularly gonorrhea or syphilis.
- Hair follicles for nits (ova) at base of hair shaft

TESTS AND PROCEDURES

- Louse or nit may be examined under microscope
- Home testing:
  - ▶ Parents can be instructed how to examine all family members for infestation.
  - ▶ Schools should perform examinations during epidemics.

 Treatment

GENERAL MEASURES

- Head lice:
  - ▶ Treat all infested household members.
  - ▶ Wash bedding, clothes, and cloth toys in hot water.
  - ▶ Treat combs by washing in hot water and soaking in medication.
  - ▶ Seal anything not washable in plastic bags for 10 to 14 days.
  - ▶ Nit removal is not necessary, especially if medication is reapplied 1 week later; if nit removal is desired, soak hair with white vinegar for 30 to 60 minutes.

Lice

- Body lice:
  - Medication is not necessary (insects live in clothing).
  - Improve hygiene.
  - Wash clothing and bedding in hot water.
  - Dry cleaning is effective, as is hot ironing (particularly along seams of clothing).
- Pubic lice:
  - Treat sexual partners to prevent reinfestation.
  - Petrolatum ointment applied to lashes 3–4 times per day for 8 to 10 days
  - Removal of nits with fine-toothed comb helpful

ACTIVITY

N/A

DIET

N/A

 ## Medications

COMMONLY PRESCRIBED DRUGS

- Permethrin (Nix)
- Pyrethrins (RID, A-200)
- Lindane (Kwell)
- Malathion (Ovide) 0.5%
- Cortisone creams
- Antibiotics for infected lesions

 ## Follow-Up

WHAT TO EXPECT

- Risk of transmission is reduced promptly after a single application of medication, so the child should be allowed to return to school or day care.
- Itching may persist for 2 weeks after therapy.
- Prognosis is excellent.

SIGNS TO WATCH

Recurrence of symptoms

PREVENTION

Head lice is not preventable.

Common Questions and Answers

Q: Did my child get head lice because my house or my child is not clean enough?
A: No, head lice are unrelated to personal hygiene. Some experts even believe lice prefer a clean scalp.

Q: Should I cut my child's long hair to get the lice out?
A: No, meticulous application of medication to the entire scalp and then pulling the medication through all hair shafts is adequate treatment. Urgently cutting a child's hair to alleviate parental anxiety can be traumatizing to the child.

Q: Can infants become infested with pubic lice?
A: Yes. Although the primary mode of transmission of the crab louse is via sexual contact, it can be transmitted through close personal contact with an infested individual. Small children become infested with crab lice on the eyebrows or lashes. The pubic louse has a predilection for the pubic and perianal area, but it can infect many hairy areas, including the armpit, the eyebrows and lashes, the beard, and the scalp.

Q: If children are infested with the head louse, how can items such as stuffed animals or other cloth toys be decontaminated?
A: Machine-washable items can be washed in hot water at temperatures of approximately 265°F. An alternative method of decontamination is sealing the items in a plastic bag for 10 days.

Q: Is removal of nits necessary to prevent spread?
A: No. They can be removed from a cosmetic standpoint by using a fine-toothed comb or by soaking the hair in a solution of white vinegar followed by wrapping the head with a towel soaked in the same solution for 30 to 60 minutes.

Q: What is appropriate treatment of infestation of the eyelashes?
A: A petroleum-based ointment should be applied 3–4 times daily for a period of 10 days. Nits should be removed from the lashes.

Light Sensitivity

 Basics

DESCRIPTION

Light sensitivity, also called sun poisoning, is a skin rash induced by exposure to sunlight. It is often a side effect of medication.

SIGNS AND SYMPTOMS

- Reddening
- Rash
- Blisters
- Usually develops shortly after sun exposure
- Pain
- Itching

CAUSES

- Sunlight
- Phenothiazines
- Diuretics
- Tetracyclines
- Sulfonamides
- Oral contraceptives
- Topicals: psoralens, coal tars, photoactive dyes (eosin, acridine orange)

SCOPE

Varies depending on cause

 Diagnosis

QUESTIONS THE DOCTOR MAY ASK

- Any oral medications?
- Any new topical agents (perfumes, lemons, limes, sunscreens)?
- Age of onset of rash?
- Occurrence in spring and summer?
- Occurrence after sun exposure?
- How long after sun exposure?

WHAT THE DOCTOR LOOKS FOR

- Physical examination
- Increased rash on nose, cheeks and forehead
- Congenital anomalies
- Evidence of arthritis or other connective tissue disease

TESTS AND PROCEDURES

- Phototesting
- Photopatch testing
- Blood tests

Treatment

GENERAL MEASURES

- Protection against sun exposure is necessary. Avoiding the sun, particularly between 10 a.m. and 2 p.m., and wearing protective clothing is important.
- Sunscreens are helpful for those sensitive to ultraviolet light. They should be waterproof and reapplied every 2 hours. The higher the sun protection factor (SPF) the better.
- Although sunscreens are less effective against blocking ultraviolet A rays (UVA) and therefore less effective in helping patients with sensitivities to longer wavelengths, Shade UVA Guard offers better protection than most.
- Opaque formulations such as zinc oxide and titanium oxide block ultraviolet and visible light but are cosmetically unacceptable. Patients with severe photosensitivities may have to avoid any significant light exposure.
- Removal of the offending agent is necessary in chemically induced light sensitivities.

ACTIVITIES

N/A

DIET

N/A

Medications

COMMONLY PRESCRIBED DRUGS

- Prednisone
- Antimalarial drugs

Follow-Up

WHAT TO EXPECT

- The outcome is variable, depending on the specific condition.

- With the exception of chemically induced photosensitivities, most of the conditions are chronic.

Common Questions and Answers

Q: What is the best sunscreen to use?
A: It depends on your particular problem. If you are sensitive to UVB, use a sunscreen with the highest SPF. If you are sensitive to UVA, Shade UVA Guard is the best.

Q: Is it true that sunscreens with an SPF above 15 are not necessary.?
A: This is definitely not true for patients with photosensitivities who have abnormal responses to light and require excessive protection. Even for the normal person, it is often not true. An SPF of 15 suggests that someone may receive 15 times more sun exposure with the sunscreen applied than without and not become sunburned. Some physicians have suggested that this protection is more than anyone should need. However, this number is calculated by testing in a controlled laboratory. Normal outdoor conditions, such as wind, reflection from water and sand, perspiration, and water exposure can significantly decrease the effectiveness of the sunscreen.

Q: What is "sun allergy"?
A: This is a lay term for light eruption, one of the most common light sensitivities presenting with pimples, vesicles, and plaques 1–2 days after sun exposure. It usually recurs every spring and most patients learn to avoid sun exposure. Ironically, it can improve with slow gradual sun exposure.

Q: Can I become allergic to sunscreens?
A: Certain active agents in sunscreens can produce an allergic response in rare individuals. If the rash recurs with each use, switch to another sunscreen with different ingredients. If the problem continues, it is necessary to consult a specialist for evaluation.

Lyme Disease

 Basics

DESCRIPTION

Lyme disease is a multisystem infection caused by a microbe transmitted by deer ticks. The disease may result in chronic arthritis and other complications.

Stage 1 includes a characteristic expanding ring-like skin rash and flu-like symptoms.

Stage 2 may involve one or more organ systems; neurologic and cardiac disease are most common.

Stage 3, chronic Lyme disease, involves arthritis and chronic neurologic symptoms.

SIGNS AND SYMPTOMS

- Stage 1:
  - ▶ Rash starts as red raised lesion
  - ▶ Expanding bull's-eye rash
  - ▶ Fever
  - ▶ Headache
  - ▶ Muscle and joint pain
  - ▶ May be no symptoms
- Stage 2:
  - ▶ Multiple ring-like rashes
  - ▶ Inflammation of facial nerves
  - ▶ Meningitis
  - ▶ Heart disorders
  - ▶ Inflammation of the testicles or liver
  - ▶ Arthritis
- Stage 3:
  - ▶ Recurring joint and muscle inflammation
  - ▶ Brain disorders (psychosis, dementia, memory loss, depression, stroke-like symptoms)
  - ▶ Nerve disorders
  - ▶ Eye disorders

CAUSES

Infection with the bacterium *Borrelia burgdorferi*, transmitted by the bite of deer tick

SCOPE

- Lyme disease can affect people of all ages, but one-third to one-half of all cases occur in children and adolescents.
- Lyme disease has now become the most common tick-borne disease in the United States, with over 8000 cases each year.
- Onset is most often in the summer months, and the endemic areas are in the northeast, north-central, and Pacific coast states.

 Diagnosis

QUESTIONS THE DOCTOR MAY ASK

- History of tick bite?
- Travel to endemic area?
- Symptoms of fever, rash or joint pain?

WHAT THE DOCTOR LOOKS FOR

- History of a tick bite can only be elicited in one-third of patients with Lyme disease.
- 50–80% have or recall having the typical rash, which is not painful or itchy, but does feel warm.
- Later, they may report swollen, painful joints or memory problems.
- The rash is very characteristic of Lyme disease. If the patient does not have the rash, there is no physical finding that gives a definite diagnosis of Lyme.
- The physical examination may be completely normal early in the course of the disease.
- The patient may have arthritis, a cranial nerve palsy, or an irregular heart beat.

TESTS AND PROCEDURES

Blood tests

Treatment

GENERAL MEASURES

Initial therapy for early Lyme disease consists of oral antibiotics.

ACTIVITY

N/A

DIET

N/A

 ## Medications

COMMONLY PRESCRIBED DRUGS

Doxycycline, tetracycline (for children over eight years), amoxicillin, erythromycin, ceftriaxone

 ## Follow-Up

WHAT TO EXPECT

- In general, the outcome for children with Lyme disease is much better than that for adults.
- Only 2% of children have chronic arthritis at 6 months after treatment.

SIGNS TO WATCH

N/A

PREVENTION

Use of topical insect repellent effective against ticks

 ## Common Questions and Answers

Q: What does the deer tick look like?
A: The deer tick is flat, very small (about the size of a pin head), and has eight legs. The adult male is black and the female is red and black. They can grow to 3 times their normal size when they are engorged with blood.

Q: Do all bites from infected deer ticks cause Lyme disease?
A: No. Even infected ticks do not cause Lyme disease if they are attached to the skin for a short period of time. If the tick is attached for less than 12 hours, the chances of transmitting the disease are very low. The longer the tick is attached, the higher the probability of disease transmission.

Measles

 Basics

DESCRIPTION

Measles is caused by a virus and is characterized by a skin eruption with a relatively predictable course. The illness involves fever, cough, conjunctivitis (pink eye), or runny nose with a rash, which has a characteristic progression.

SIGNS AND SYMPTOMS

- Before the illness, white spots may appear on the inner surface of the cheek.
- A generalized rash lasting 3 days or longer
- A temperature of 101°F or higher *and* cough, runny nose, or conjunctivitis
- The rash appears on the face (often the nape of the neck, initially) and abdomen 14 days after exposure to measles virus.
- The rash spreads from the head to the feet.
- After 3 to 4 days, the rash begins to clear, leaving a brownish discoloration and flaking skin.
- Fever usually resolves by the fourth day of rash.
- Sore throat and swollen lymph nodes in neck

CAUSES

Infection by the measles virus

SCOPE

- Measles is a highly contagious disease.
- Transmission of measles is thought to be mainly airborne.
- Hospital or clinic waiting rooms (especially pediatric emergency department waiting rooms) have been identified as a major risk, accounting for up to 45% of the known exposures in this setting.
- In 1983, there were only 0.7 cases per 100,000 population. In 1990, however, 27,672 cases were reported with 89 deaths.
- The reason for the 1989–1991 outbreak was failure to adequately vaccinate preschool-aged children.
- Patients are contagious from 1 to 2 days *before* onset of symptoms until 5 days after the appearance of the rash.
- The incubation period is generally 8 to 12 days from exposure to onset of symptoms and approximately 14 days until the appearance of rash.

Diagnosis

QUESTIONS THE DOCTOR MAY ASK

- Exposure to measles?
- Immunization history?
- Presence of cough, running nose, or red eye?
- Progression of rash?

WHAT THE DOCTOR LOOKS FOR

- Characteristic signs and symptoms of measles
- White spot on inside of cheek

TESTS AND PROCEDURES

- Virus may be cultured and/or identified.
- Blood tests

 ## Treatment

GENERAL MEASURES

- There is no specific therapy for this infection other than supportive care.
- Fever-reducing medications, plenty of oral fluids, and room humidification to help reduce cough are usually all that is needed.
- All suspected cases of measles should be reported immediately to the health department.

ACTIVITY

Any person suspected of having measles should be in respiratory isolation.

DIET

N/A

 ## Medications

COMMONLY PRESCRIBED MEDICATION

- Antifever remedies
- Vitamin A for children 6 to 24 months old

 ## Follow-Up

WHAT TO EXPECT

- In uncomplicated measles infection, the patient begins feeling better with a fading of rash on the third and fourth day.
- Mortality in the 1989–90 outbreak occurred in 3 of every 1000 cases in the United States.
- Mortality rates are higher in immunocompromised children.

PREVENTION

- Routine vaccination against measles, mumps, rubella (MMR)
- With the recent resurgence of measles, aggressive employee immunization programs should be pursued for all health care workers.

 ## Common Questions and Answers

Q: How long is incubation period?
A: 10 days; range 8–22 days.

Q: Is one measles immunization satisfactory?
A: No. A second dose should be given at 11–12 years.

Meningitis

 ## Basics

DESCRIPTION

Meningitis is inflammation of the membranes of the brain or spinal cord usually caused by bacteria, viruses, fungi, and (rarely) parasites. It can result in death, seizures, deafness, and other serious neurologic consequences.

SIGNS AND SYMPTOMS:

- Irritability, crying
- Loss of appetite
- Nausea and vomiting
- Stiff neck in toddlers and children
- Pain on flexing the neck
- Bulging soft spot (fontanelle)

CAUSES

Infection by bacteria, virus, fungus, or other organism

SCOPE

- Most bacterial meningitis (80%) occurs in patients less than 24 months of age.
- 85% of viral meningitis tends to occur in outbreaks in summer and early fall.
- Meningitis caused by Candida (a fungus) occurs in ill premature infants and others with an impaired immune system.
- The incidence of disease due to *Mycobacteria tuberculosis,* which causes tuberculosis (TB), is on the rise throughout the world.
- TB meningitis occurs in 1 of every 300 primary TB infections.
- TB meningitis is most commonly seen in children ages 6 months to 6 years of age.
- Cryptococcus is a fungus-like organism that can affect the lungs, bone, internal organs, skin, and brain.

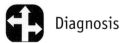 ## Diagnosis

QUESTIONS THE DOCTOR MAY ASK

- Fever?
- Contacts?
- Travel?

WHAT THE DOCTOR LOOKS FOR

- Signs and symptoms of meningitis
- Common chief complaints by the infant's caretakers include:
  - ▶ Irritable or "sleeping all the time"
  - ▶ "Won't take to bottle"
  - ▶ "Not acting right"
  - ▶ "Cries when moved or picked up"
  - ▶ "Won't stop crying"
  - ▶ "Soft spot bulging out"
- Cryptococcus:
  - ▶ Headache
  - ▶ Fever
  - ▶ Neurologic symptoms: hearing impairment, double vision, confusion, lethargy
- Stiff neck
- Rash
- Muscle tone, weakness
- Abnormal eye movements

TESTS AND PROCEDURES

- Blood tests
- Lumbar puncture (spinal tap)
- Cultures and other microbiological tests
- Arterial blood gasses

 ## Treatment

GENERAL MEASURES

- Hospitalization is required.
- Assure adequate ventilation, hydration, and supportive care.
- Intravenous fluids and medications
- Blood transfusion may be needed.

ACTIVITY

N/A

DIET

N/A

Medications

COMMONLY PRESCRIBED DRUGS

- Antimicrobial agents: ampicillin, cefotaxime IV, vancomycin, cefotaxime
- Amphotericin, 5-fluorocytosine, fluconazole
- Isoniazid, rifampin, pyrazinamide, ethambutol, streptomycin
- Acyclovir

Follow-Up

WHAT TO EXPECT

- Most children with bacterial meningitis break the fever by 7 to 10 days after starting therapy with gradual improvement in activity and less irritability.
- Evaluation for neurologic damage, such as hearing and vision testing, is essential.
- Preventive medication for patient and family before discharge
- Bacterial meningitis:
  - ▶ Approximately 1500 deaths each year
  - ▶ Lasting effects of the infection, including hearing deficits and neurologic damage, may occur in up to 25% of children.

- Viral meningitis: Prognosis for viral meningitis is good.
- Lyme disease: Prognosis with diagnosis and treatment is good.
- Tuberculous meningitis:
  - ▶ The long-term prognosis in children with tuberculous meningitis depends on the stage of disease in which treatment is begun.
  - ▶ Complete recovery occurs in 94% of those whose treatment starts early, but only 18–50% for those whose treatment starts in the later stages of disease
- Prognosis for cryptococcus is good with treatment.

SIGNS TO WATCH

N/A

PREVENTION

- The *Haemophilus influenzae* type b (HIB) vaccine has markedly reduced the incidence of meningitis and other invasive HIB infections.
- Preventive treatment with rifampin (antiviral drug)

Common Questions and Answers

Q: What are sources of cryptococcus in nature?
A: Pigeon droppings and soil.

Meningococcemia

Basics

DESCRIPTION

Meningococcemia is a systemic infection with the bacterium *Neisseria meningitides*. Widespread disease occurs when the organism penetrates the nasal passages and enters the bloodstream, where it replicates. Complications include inflammation of the covering of the brain, inflammation of the heart, bleeding, arthritis, and pneumonia. It results in deafness in 5 to 10% of survivors.

SIGNS AND SYMPTOMS

- Rash
- Irritability, crying
- Loss of appetite
- Nausea and vomiting
- Stiff neck
- Pain on flexing the neck
- Bulging soft spot (fontanelle)

CAUSES

Bacterial infection

SCOPE

- Children less than age 5 are most often affected.
- During epidemics, relatively more school-age children may be affected.
- The disease occurs most commonly in winter and spring months.
- Increased disease activity may follow an influenza outbreak.

Diagnosis

QUESTIONS THE DOCTOR MAY ASK

- Onset of fever, ill-feeling and rash?
- Exposure to others with illness?

WHAT THE DOCTOR LOOKS FOR

- Time of onset of fever, malaise, and rash
- Recognition of abnormal vital signs and lethargy
- Careful examination of the skin for minute bleeding
- Stiff neck that is painful when flexed
- Signs and symptoms of meningitis

TESTS AND PROCEDURES

- Culture of organism from blood, spinal fluid, and skin lesions
- Urinalysis
- Blood tests

Treatment

GENERAL MEASURES

- Close monitoring of vital signs and clinical status should follow, preferably in an intensive care setting.
- Hospitalized patients require respiratory isolation until 24 hours after appropriate antibiotic therapy.
- Treatment of exposed contacts, including household, day care, and nursery school

ACTIVITY

N/A

DIET

N/A

 ## Medications

COMMONLY PRESCRIBED DRUGS

- Antibiotics: penicillin, cefotaxime, ceftriaxone, third-generation cephalosporins, chloramphenicol
- Rifampin for family and contacts of patient.

 ## Follow-Up

WHAT TO EXPECT

- Fatality rate of meningococcemia is 20%, even when recognized and treated.
- Fatality rate of meningococcal meningitis is 5%.
- The most severe cases often have a rapid progression from onset of symptoms to death over a matter of hours.

SIGNS TO WATCH

N/A

PREVENTION

Vaccination

 ## Common Questions and Answers

Q: When is meningococcal vaccine indicated?
A: In immune compromised patients without spleens and in epidemics in conjunction with Rifampin.

Menstrual Disorders

 Basics

DESCRIPTION

Dysmenorrhea is pain associated with menstrual flow characterized by lower abdominal cramping with radiation to the back and thighs.

SIGNS AND SYMPTOMS

- Pain
- Interference with everyday activities
- Nausea and vomiting
- Fatigue
- Nervousness
- Dizziness
- Diarrhea
- Backache
- Headache

CAUSES

Thought to be due to uterine contractions combined with an excess of hormone

SCOPE

- 45–60% of all women have some degree of dysmenorrhea.
- 10% of these women are incapacitated for 1 to 3 days a month.
- 38–66% of adolescents experience dysmenorrhea.

 Diagnosis

QUESTIONS THE DOCTOR MAY ASK

- How bad are the cramps?
- Do the cramps interfere with going to school or other activities?
- Are there other symptoms that accompany the cramps?
- Menstrual history?
- Sexual history?
- Gastrointestinal and genitourinary history?

WHAT THE DOCTOR LOOKS FOR

- Physical examination
- Palpation of uterus

TESTS AND PROCEDURES

- Blood tests
- Culture of reproductive tract for microbiologic analysis

Treatment

GENERAL MEASURES

Education and reassurance

ACTIVITY

Exercise

DIET

Avoid high-salt diet and caffeine.

 Medications

COMMONLY PRESCRIBED DRUGS

- Aspirin, acetaminophen, ibuprofen, naproxen sodium
- Oral contraceptive pills provide both contraception and relief from primary dysmenorrhea.
- Tolmetin (Tolectin)
- Sulindac (Clinoril)
- Mefenamic acid (Ponstel)
- Meclofenamate (Meclomen)

 Follow-Up

WHAT TO EXPECT

- Should see improvement within 3 to 4 menstrual cycles
- Dysmenorrhea often lessens in the mid-to-late 20s.

SIGNS TO WATCH

- Gastrointestinal distress
- No response to medical management. Referral to gynecologist for laparascopic evaluation should be strongly considered.

PREVENTION

N/A

 Common Questions and Answers

Q: When should I consider oral contraceptive pills for a patient with dysmenorrhea?
A: If the patient has Grade II or higher dysmenorrhea that is not responding to medication, or if she has many systemic symptoms. Oral contraceptives should also be suggested to sexually active adolescents with all grades of dysmenorrhea. The advantages are lessening of dysmenorrhea, less menstrual flow, and less iron-deficiency anemia.

Q: How do I distinguish primary from secondary dysmenorrhea?
A: Primary amenorrhea usually begins gradually 2-4 years after the onset of menses. In contrast, an adolescent with isolated atypical, painful, menstrual periods should be evaluated for complications of pregnancy and/or genital tract infections. The older adolescent with a long history of increasingly painful menstrual periods should be evaluated for endometriosis. Congenital malformations of the genital tract are very rare and usually cause severe pain with the first menstrual period, unlike primary dysmenorrhea and endometriosis. Most malformations that cause dysmenorrhea include some blood flow outlet obstruction, and pelvic masses are often detected by examination or ultrasound.

Q: What are the characteristics of endometriosis in adolescents?
A: Adolescents with endometriosis often display dysmenorrhea of increasing severity. Other symptoms include abnormal vaginal bleeding, dyspareunia, and intestinal and bladder dysfunction. They may have no findings on pelvic examination, but some display posterior cul de sac tenderness and a smaller percentage display posterior cul de sac nodularity. The diagnosis is best made by laparascopic evaluation.

Mental Retardation

 Basics

DESCRIPTION

Mental retardation is a nonprogressive impairment of cognitive development with significantly below-average intellectual function (IQ less than 70) associated with impairments in behavior and manifested during the developmental period (age less than 18 years).

- Mental retardation implies permanent intellectual disability and is usually described as mild, moderate, severe, and profound. A recent proposal reduces the definition to two levels, mild and severe.
- Mental deficiency in children more commonly results from disorders reflecting abnormal brain development during the pregnancy, birth, or early infancy.
- Mental retardation is associated with numerous other conditions, including cerebral palsy, blindness, and other disturbances.

CAUSES

- Genetic disorders
- Abnormal brain development
- Infections
- Substances that cause birth defects (alcohol, cocaine, other medications)
- Vascular disorders during pregnancy (stroke)
- Complications of prematurity
- Metabolic disorders
- Trauma (complications of delivery)
- Neonatal asphyxia
- Blood disorders
- Other disorders

SCOPE

- Mental retardation affects 2–3% of the child population in the United States, with the peak age at diagnosis 10–14 years.
- Children with mild mental retardation are diagnosed at a significantly later age than those with severe retardation.
- Most children classified as retarded are in the mild range.
- More common in males

 Diagnosis

QUESTIONS THE DOCTOR MAY ASK

- Maternal health?
- Exposures?
- Infections?
- Perinatal history?
- Developmental history?

WHAT THE DOCTOR LOOKS FOR

- Physical examination
- Head size
- Eye exam
- Physical anomalies
- Skin examination

TESTS AND PROCEDURES

- Blood tests
- Urinalysis
- Genetic analysis
- Hearing and vision, visual screening
- Neuropsychological evaluation
- Electroencephalogram (EEG)
- Neurologic testing
- Developmental testing
- Magnetic resonance imaging (MRI) of brain

Treatment

GENERAL MEASURES

- Consultations with child development, genetics, neurology, and metabolic specialists as appropriate
- Developmental assessment and psychological testing to identify functional levels and areas of strengths should be carried out.
- Early intervention should be initiated and programs reassessed at regular intervals by multidisciplinary teams to meet the needs of the child.
- Nutritional intervention is critical for the many genetic defects in metabolism that can cause mental retardation.
- Treatment of hydrocephalus, if present

ACTIVITY

N/A

DIET

N/A

 ## Medications

COMMONLY PRESCRIBED DRUGS

- Medication for seizures, if needed
- Chelation therapy for lead poisoning, if needed
- Thyroid replacement therapy for hypothyroidism, if needed

 ## Follow-Up

WHAT TO EXPECT

- General pediatric care and treatment of associated impairments
- Early intervention and reassessment of educational programs as the child ages and needs change
- Genetic counseling to address recurrence risks for the family
- Transition to adulthood regarding living situation, job placement, and sexuality

 ## Common Questions and Answers

Q: When can you make a diagnosis of mental retardation?
A: The severity of cognitive impairment determines when the diagnosis is made. In a severely retarded child, the diagnosis is usually apparent by age 2. In a mildly affected child, the diagnosis often is delayed to an older age.

Q: What is the prognosis in a child with mental retardation?
A: Although the answer depends on the severity of the retardation and the presence of associated defects, diagnosis of mental retardation implies that the clinician foresees significant permanent mental handicap.

Mesenteric Adenitis

 Basics

DESCRIPTION

Mesenteric adenitis is a self-limiting inflammation of lymph nodes in the mesentery, a structure adjacent to the intestines.

SIGNS AND SYMPTOMS

- Abdominal pain
- Tenderness of the abdomen
- Pain may initially be in the upper abdomen, right lower quadrant, or generalized.
- Between spasms, the patient feels well and can walk without any difficulty.
- Nausea and vomiting
- Flushed skin
- Fever

CAUSES

- Viral infection
- Allergic reaction to a foreign protein

SCOPE

- Most common cause of acute abdominal pain in young adults and children
- True incidence is not known.
- Most common in patients under 18 years of age
- May have a history of recent sore throat or upper respiratory tract infection

 Diagnosis

QUESTIONS THE DOCTOR MAY ASK

- Fever?
- Pain in abdomen?
- Loss of appetite?

WHAT THE DOCTOR LOOKS FOR

- Abdominal pain
- Infection of throat
- Swollen glands in neck
- May appear similar to appendicitis

TESTS AND PROCEDURES

- Blood tests
- Abdominal ultrasound
- Upper gastrointestinal (GI) series

Treatment

GENERAL MEASURES

Mainly supportive

ACTIVITY

N/A

DIET

N/A

 ## Follow-Up

WHAT TO EXPECT

- Acute symptoms may take days to resolve and generally last a few days after the associated viral symptoms have resolved.
- Prognosis is very good; most patients recover completely without any specific treatment.
- Death is very rare and may only occur when secondary bacterial infection develops.

SIGNS TO WATCH

Increasing abdominal pain; vomiting; fever; toxic appearance; severe, persistent tenderness

PREVENTION

N/A

 ## Common Questions and Answers

Q: Can one differentiate between acute appendicitis and nonspecific mesenteric adenitis?
A: Patients with mesenteric adenitis cannot localize the exact point of the most intense pain, unlike appendicitis. Between spasms, patients with nonspecific mesenteric adenitis feel well and can walk without any difficulty.

Migraine

Basics

DESCRIPTION

Migraine is an attack of headache lasting 4–72 hours. Episodes vary from more than once a week to less than one per year, with symptoms abating completely between attacks. Nonspecific symptoms may be felt hours to days before headache.

SIGNS AND SYMPTOMS

- Four main types
  - ▶ Classic migraine
  - ▶ Common migraine
  - ▶ Complicated migraine
  - ▶ Migraine variants
- Symptoms of migraine vary from person to person or from attack to attack within the same individual.
- Five phases of a classic migraine:
  - ▶ Prodrome: Warning signs preceding migraine include mood disruptions (e.g., euphoria, irritability, depression), fatigue, muscle tension, food craving, bloating, yawning.
  - ▶ Aura: The aura consists of visual disruptions, including spots, geometric patterns, and occasionally hallucinations. Headache typically begins within 1 hour after aura.
  - ▶ Headache: one-sided, throbbing pain of 4 to 72 hours duration, intensified by movement; nausea, vomiting, diarrhea, light sensitivity, sound sensitivity, muscle tenderness, lightheadedness, and dizziness
  - ▶ Headache termination: Without treatment, termination usually occurs with sleep.
  - ▶ Postdrome: Headache pain has resolved but other symptoms linger, such as food intolerance, impaired concentration, fatigue, and muscle soreness.
- Common migraine does not have visual prodrome.
- Complicated migraine may have loss of vision, weakness on one side or loss of speech.
- Variants include dizziness and vomiting.

CAUSES

Exact cause is often unknown, but may be due to numerous factors. A family history is common (found in 60% of individuals who have migraines).

SCOPE

- Migraine occurs in 3 to 5% of children before puberty and increases to 10 to 20% during the 20s.
- Female:male ratio is equal before puberty and increases 2:1 after puberty.

Diagnosis

QUESTIONS THE DOCTOR MAY ASK

- Family history?
- Warning signs?
- Visual changes?
- Location of headache?
- Description of stress?

WHAT THE DOCTOR LOOKS FOR

- Neurologic signs
- Eye examination
- Jaw pain
- Muscle tension

TESTS AND PROCEDURES

- Blood tests
- X-rays of head
- Computed tomography (CT), magnetic resonance imaging (MRI)
- Electroencephalogram (EEG)
- Spinal tap

Treatment

GENERAL MEASURES

- Compression to temple artery or tender areas of scalp or neck on affected side
- Cold compresses to area of pain
- Rest with pillows comfortably supporting head or neck in quiet, darkened area
- Withdrawal from stressful surroundings
- Sleep
- Biofeedback and early psychologic intervention in appropriate cases or when pain behaviors are first identified
- Most attacks of migraine are managed with self-care.

ACTIVITY

N/A

DIET

N/A

 Medications

COMMONLY PRESCRIBED DRUGS

- Sumatriptan (Imitrex)
- Dihydroergotamine (DHE), metoclopramide, prochlorperazine
- Ergotamine-caffeine (Cafergot)
- Aspirin
- Acetaminophen
- Ibuprofen (Nuprin, Motrin)
- Naproxen (Naprosyn)
- Ketoprofen (Orudis)
- Ketorolac (Toradol)
- Isometheptene-dichloralphenazone-acetaminophen (Midrin)
- Acetaminophen-butalbital (Phrenilin)
- Acetaminophen-butalbital (Fioricet), acetaminophen-butalbital-codeine (Fiorinal)
- Butorphanol (Stadol)
- Zolmitriptan, naratriptan, eletriptan, rizatriptan
- Propranolol (Inderal)
- Atenolol (Tenormin)
- Nadolol (Corgard)
- Timolol (Blocadren)
- Metoprolol (Lopressor)
- Amitriptyline (Elavil)
- Nortriptyline (Pamelor)
- Verapamil (Calan, Isoptin)
- Isradipine (DynaCirc)
- Methysergide (Sansert)
- Cyproheptadine (Periactin)
- Valproic acid (Depakene) or divalproex (Depakote)

 Follow-Up

WHAT TO EXPECT

N/A

SIGNS TO WATCH

N/A

PREVENTION

- Avoid triggers of attacks.
- Biofeedback and psychologic intervention may be helpful.
- Preventive therapy: If attacks significantly interfere with lifestyle or are not adequately controlled, daily preventive therapy may be appropriate.
- A referral to a specialist may be helpful in difficult cases that do not respond to treatment.

 Common Questions and Answers

Q: When should migraine be treated?
A: Many children with migraine headaches have attacks so infrequently that preventive treatment is not necessary. Treatment should be considered when attacks occur at least once a month.

Q: What about allergy and headache?
A: Many believe that headache represents a symptom of allergies.

Q: At what age may migraine begin?
A: Even 2–3 year olds may have symptoms of migraine.

Milia

 ## Basics

DESCRIPTION

Milia are raised white rashes that occur commonly and spontaneously on the face and trunk.

SIGNS AND SYMPTOMS

- 1- to 2-millimeter bright white lesions with smooth surface, most often found on cheeks, nose, chin, forehead, but occasionally on the back of the of hands and over knees, especially if related to trauma
- Occasionally, lesions may be seen on upper trunk, extremities, penis, or mucous membranes.

CAUSES

Retention of keratin and sebaceous material within the hair follicle of the newborn

SCOPE

Up to 40% of newborns have milia on the skin; in older patients, most often related to trauma or healing blister

 ## Diagnosis

QUESTIONS THE DOCTOR MAY ASK

- History of atopy and/or allergic conjunctivitis?
- Absence of itching?
- Trauma?

WHAT THE DOCTOR LOOKS FOR

- Typical lesions of milia

Treatment

GENERAL MEASURES

- No need for treatment in infants because milia are benign, symptom-free, and often resolve on their own.
- May be removed by minor surgical procedure

ACTIVITY

N/A

DIET

N/A

 ## Medications

COMMONLY PRESCRIBED DRUGS

N/A

 ## Follow-Up

WHAT TO EXPECT

- Without treatment, most lesions resolve in 1 to 2 weeks.
- Lesions may recur with trauma or re-eruption of blistering disease.

SIGNS TO WATCH

Persistence of symptoms

PREVENTION

N/A

 ## Common Questions and Answers

Q: Will the lesions get bigger before they go away?
A: No, there is no tendency to enlarge with time.

Milk Protein Allergy

Basics

DESCRIPTION

Milk protein allergy describes symptoms affecting the gastrointestinal tract, skin, and respiratory tract that result from ingesting cow's milk protein. Predisposing factors include age under 2 years, early milk feeding, and a history of allergies.

SIGNS AND SYMPTOMS

- Failure to thrive
- Chronic diarrhea
- May be bloody diarrhea
- Vomiting
- Abdominal distention
- Anemia
- Rectal bleeding

CAUSES

Allergy to cow proteins found in milk

SCOPE

Milk protein allergy is estimated to affect 2–7.5% of otherwise normal children

Diagnosis

QUESTIONS THE DOCTOR MAY ASK

N/A

WHAT THE DOCTOR LOOKS FOR

Signs and symptoms of milk protein allergy

TESTS AND PROCEDURES

- Blood tests
- Stool analysis
- Endoscopy

Treatment

GENERAL MEASURES

- Removal of cow's milk protein-containing products from the diet is the focus.
- Because approximately 10–30% of children allergic to cow's milk may also be allergic to soy, hydrolyzed formulas (Pregestimil/Nutramigen/Alimentum) are the formulas used for cow's milk protein intolerance.

ACTIVITY

N/A

DIET

See General measures

Medications

COMMONLY PRESCRIBED DRUGS

N/A

 ## Follow-Up

WHAT TO EXPECT

- Resolution of bloody stools usually occurs within 24 to 72 hours after cow's milk is stopped.
- Tolerance to cow's milk protein usually develops between the ages of 1 and 2 years, and re-introduction of a normal diet can be safely done at that time.
- Symptoms of intolerance may persist past the third year of life, and approximately 20% have symptoms that persist to 6 years of age.
- With a history of severe allergic reaction, the cow's milk challenge should be done in a hospital under medical supervision.

SIGNS TO WATCH

N/A

PREVENTION

N/A

 ## Common Questions and Answers

Q: How long will my child be allergic to cow's milk?
A: Tolerance usually develops between 1 and 2 years of age; however, in 20% of these children, symptoms may persist to the age of 6.

Mononucleosis

 Basics

DESCRIPTION

Mononucleosis, or "mono," is a viral illness caused by the Epstein-Barr virus (EBV). The illness is characterized by fatigue, fever, enlarged spleen, enlarged lymph nodes, and sore throat.

SIGNS AND SYMPTOMS

- Malaise
- Fatigue
- Headache
- Fever
- Enlarged lymph nodes
- Tonsillitis
- Swelling around eyes
- Rash

CAUSES

Epstein-Barr virus

SCOPE

- EBV spreads between individuals via saliva and occasionally via blood transfusions.
- Almost all adults have been exposed to EBV.
- Children who live in areas where the population is dense or who have a low socioeconomic status usually become affected within the first 3 years of life.

 Diagnosis

QUESTIONS THE DOCTOR MAY ASK

N/A

WHAT THE DOCTOR LOOKS FOR

- Incubation period 30–50 days
- A prodrome period before illness marked by malaise and fever lasting 2–5 days
- Young children are more likely to have a rash or abdominal pain.
- Large spleen
- Rash
- Large tonsils
- Tiredness, malaise, loss of appetite, sore throat, swollen glands

TESTS AND PROCEDURES

- Blood tests
- Identification of virus

 Treatment

GENERAL MEASURES

Supportive care and symptomatic treatment are sufficient for most cases.

ACTIVITY

See Common questions and answers

DIET

N/A

Medications

COMMONLY PRESCRIBED DRUGS

- Acetaminophen or ibuprofen reduce fever and provide analgesia.
- Oral, and sometimes intravenous, rehydration is often indicated.
- Corticosteroids (prednisone) for large tonsils that interfere with breathing.

 ## Follow-Up

WHAT TO EXPECT

- Most patients with EBV infection will recover uneventfully in 1 to 4 weeks.
- Recovery often follows a course of improvement and a worsening of symptoms.
- The spleen may remain enlarged for weeks after infection.
- Fatigue may persist months after recovery.
- Long-lasting immunity generally ensues.
- Prognosis of patients with unusual manifestations of EBV infection depends on the severity of the illness and the organ system involved.

SIGNS TO WATCH

- Abdominal pain
- Trauma to large spleen
- Increasing fatigue

PREVENTION

- No vaccine is available.
- Hospitalized patients need not be isolated when rigorous hand washing is employed.
- Avoid intimate contact with those with a compromised immune system.
- Patients with recent EBV infection, either proven or suspected, should not donate blood.

 ## Common Questions and Answers

Q: How long after infectious mononucleosis may a patient return to athletic activity?
A: Over half of patients with "mono" have an enlarged spleen that is prone to rupture. All athletic activity should be restricted until no evidence exists for a clinically enlarged or tender spleen. If this criterion is met, and the patient feels subjectively better, light (noncontact) activities may be resumed. Return to contact sports is not advised until at least 4–6 weeks after resolution of all signs and symptoms of illness. Some experts recommend ultrasound study of the spleen before return to heavy contact sports, such as rugby, football, lacrosse, and hockey.

Q: Should all patients with infectious mononucleosis be given corticosteroids?
A: Even though children may feel tired, weak, and ill, symptomatic EBV infection is most often self-limited with only symptomatic care. Long-term effects from the use of steroids to treat EBV are not known. EBV has been linked to certain lymphoproliferative disorders, and theoretical risks to modulating the host immune response with corticosteroids have been proposed.

Mumps

Basics

DESCRIPTION

Mumps is an acute viral infection that causes inflammation of one or both parotid glands, which are located just behind the corner of the jaw. The swollen parotid glands can get quite large, obscuring the normal contour of the cheek. Epidemics of mumps occur in late winter and spring. The mumps virus is transmitted through the air. Mumps may lead to secondary bacterial infection.

SIGNS AND SYMPTOMS

- Pain and swelling in one or both parotid glands at the corner of the jaw
- Pre-illness syndrome of fever, neck muscle ache, malaise
- Swelling peaks in 1 to 3 days, lasts 3–7 days.
- Sour foods cause pain.
- Moderate fever, usually not above 104°F (40.0°C)
- May affect joints, testicles (orchitis), thyroid, breasts, pancreas
- Rash
- Up to 50% of cases have no symptoms.

CAUSES

Viral infection

SCOPE

- 85% of mumps cases occur before 15 years of age, but the illness is more severe in adults; males and females are affected with equal frequency.
- Spread is via the respiratory route.
- Incidence of this once very common disease has declined dramatically since the advent of universal childhood immunization.
- Outbreaks, however, continue to occur.
- Mumps is most common in the late winter and spring.
- One attack of mumps confers lifelong immunity.

Diagnosis

QUESTIONS THE DOCTOR MAY ASK

- Does the pain (at the parotid) intensify with the tasting of sour liquids?
- Fever?
- Headache?
- Testicular pain?
- Immunization history?

WHAT THE DOCTOR LOOKS FOR

- Cannot see angle of jaw
- Ear moves forward
- Swelling of salivary duct
- Difficulty swallowing or speaking
- Testicular pain and swelling
- Physical examination

TESTS AND PROCEDURES

- Blood tests
- Lumbar puncture (spinal tap) may be done if meningitis suspected.
- Isolation and identification of mumps virus

Treatment

GENERAL MEASURES

Supportive therapy is all that is required in mumps.

ACTIVITY

N/A

DIET

N/A

 ## Medications

COMMONLY PRESCRIBED DRUGS

Antibiotics if secondary bacterial infection occurs.

 ## Follow-Up

WHAT TO EXPECT

- Most children have resolution of glandular swelling by approximately 1 week.
- Disappearance of testicular pain and swelling can be expected 4–6 days after onset.
- Testicular atrophy is common, although infertility is rare.
- Children should not return to school until at least 9 days after the onset of parotid swelling.

SIGNS TO WATCH

N/A

PREVENTION

Mumps vaccine

 ## Common Questions and Answers

Q: Should immunization be deferred in children with intercurrent illness?
A: No, children with minor illnesses, even with fever, should be vaccinated.

Q: Should vaccination be withheld in children living with immunocompromised hosts?
A: No, vaccinated children do not transmit mumps vaccine virus.

Necrotizing Enterocolitis

 ## Basics

DESCRIPTION

Necrotizing enterocolitis (NEC) is an inflammatory bowel disorder affecting the premature infant; only 10% of cases occur in full-term infants. It is the most common and most serious acquired gastrointestinal disorder among hospitalized pre-term infants and is associated with significant illness and death.

SIGNS AND SYMPTOMS

- Abdominal distention
- Bloody stools
- Vomiting

CAUSES

The cause of NEC is unknown, but it is believed to be due to multiple factors.

SCOPE

- The prevalence for NEC is approximately 4% and the incidence ranges from 1 per 2000–4000 live births.
- NEC usually has an onset within the first 2 weeks of life and after oral feeding has begun.
- The more premature the infant, the longer the child is at risk for developing NEC; cases have been reported 3 months after birth.
- The overall mortality rate for infants with NEC is between 20 and 40%.

 ## Diagnosis

QUESTIONS THE DOCTOR MAY ASK

- Lethargy
- Diarrhea
- Unstable temperature

WHAT THE DOCTOR LOOKS FOR

- Signs and symptoms of NEC
- Infants with more advanced disease may present with more serious problems.
- Abdominal distention, bloody stools, vomiting bile

TESTS AND PROCEDURES

- X-ray of abdomen
- Blood tests

Treatment

GENERAL MEASURES

- Therapy is based on the severity and progression of the symptoms.
- NEC is managed in the hospital.
- Length of therapy and reinstitution of feeds tends should be based on severity of the episode and on clinical, laboratory, and X-ray findings.
- Overall, the best therapy for NEC is prevention, using slow oral-feeding methods.

ACTIVITY

N/A

DIET

- No oral feedings
- I.V. fluids

 ## Follow-Up

WHAT TO EXPECT

- Despite early recognition and intervention, NEC is associated with significantly high rates of illness and death.
- May cause long-term effects

SIGNS TO WATCH

N/A

PREVENTION

N/A

 ## Common Questions and Answers

Q: What problems may evolve from NEC?
A: Anemia, intestinal strictures and short bowel syndrome.

Neurofibromatosis

 ## Basics

DESCRIPTION

Neurofibromatosis is a syndrome in which tumors grow along nerves. Neurologic effects include cognitive disability, tumors of the nervous system, and stroke (rare). Tumors may be cosmetically disfiguring and physically limiting.

SIGNS AND SYMPTOMS

- Café-au-lait spots (round, darkly pigmented patches of skin)
- Neurofibromas: disfiguring tumors of the skin

CAUSE

Genetic defect

SCOPE

- Neurofibromatosis affects up to 1 in every 3000–4000 live births.
- Neurofibromatosis affects 100,000 Americans.

 ## Diagnosis

QUESTIONS THE DOCTOR MAY ASK

- Visual problems?
- Seizures?
- Back pain?
- Headache?
- Lump in skin?
- History of neurofibromatosis in a first-degree relative, mother, or father?

WHAT THE DOCTOR LOOKS FOR

- Characteristic skin tumors
- Associated conditions: neurologic impairment, breathing problems
- Pain in the joints, extremities, back
- Hypertension
- Careful search for tumors
- Scoliosis

TESTS AND PROCEDURES

- DNA testing
- Kidney studies
- X-rays, magnetic resonance imaging (MRI)

Treatment

GENERAL MEASURES

- Presently, there is no treatment for tumor growth, except surgery.
- Tumors cannot be predicted based on the experience of other affected family members.
- Interventions are palliative and supportive.
- Surgery is done on those tumors that are medically compromising, painful, or cosmetically disfiguring.
- Family counseling
- Vigilance/anticipatory care regarding common psychological and developmental issues, such as speech delay, incoordination, hyperactivity/attention deficit, and learning disabilities, is necessary. Early educational assessment and interventions may improve developmental outcome.

ACTIVITY

N/A

DIET

N/A

 ## Follow-Up

WHAT TO EXPECT

- Monitoring for the development of tumors, hypertension, and psychological and developmental disabilities
- Deaths have been associated with cancer, heart disease, and strokes, similar to the general population.
- Optimism: Studies indicate that people with neurofibromatosis can live long, full lives.

SIGNS TO WATCH

- High blood pressure
- Eye examination

PREVENTION

N/A

 ## Common Questions and Answers

Q: Can neurofibromatosis develop into cancer?
A: Most tumors are benign and remain benign (even large tumors). In rare cases, they may become malignant.

Q: My child has neurofibromatosis. What specialists must he see?
A: Your child should have yearly checkups with a physician familiar with the issues of neurofibromatosis (could be a family physician, pediatrician, child neurologist, geneticist) who will know when to refer to other specialists. Otherwise, periodic visits to an ophthalmologist with experience in neurofibromatosis is the only routine recommendation.

Nosebleed

 ## Basics

DESCRIPTION

Nosebleed, or epistaxis, is a hemorrhage from the nostril, nasal cavity, or nasal portion of the throat.

SIGNS AND SYMPTOMS

Usually bleeding from the nostril. However, nose can bleed to the back of the throat and not be apparent, resulting in nausea, the spitting or vomiting of blood, or the appearance of dark, tarry stool.

CAUSES

- Unknown (most common)
- Injury: nose picking, low humidity, foreign body
- Infection
- Vascular abnormalities
- Cancer
- High blood pressure
- Blood clotting disorders
- Deviation or perforation of the nasal septum
- Allergies

SCOPE

- Nosebleeds occur in all ages throughout the year.
- Children 2–10 years of age are most commonly affected.
- Nosebleeds are more common in the winter.

 ## Diagnosis

QUESTIONS THE DOCTOR MAY ASK

- Trauma?
- Frequency of occurrence?
- Persistence of bleeding?
- Nosepicking behavior/trauma?
- Nasal congestion, discharge, obstruction?
- Allergies?
- Medications or drugs of abuse (especially cocaine)?
- Bruising or bleeding?
- Menstrual history?
- Family history of systemic disease or bleeding disorder?

WHAT THE DOCTOR LOOKS FOR

- Physical examination
- Size of bleeding
- Trauma
- Nasal polyps

TESTS AND PROCEDURES

Blood tests

 ## Treatment

GENERAL MEASURES

- Elevate the head of the bed.
- Direct pressure, applied by gently squeezing the nostrils, is usually sufficient to stop most nosebleeds.
- Nasal packing may be done.
- Parental reassurance is important.

Medications

COMMONLY PRESCRIBED DRUGS

Phenylephrine, oxymetazoline, epinephrine, cocaine

 Follow-Up

WHAT TO EXPECT

- Nosebleeds are easily controlled and self-limited in most instances.
- Families should be given instructions in basic first aid for nosebleeds caused by minor injury, such as sneezing or excessive manipulation.
- Severe or recurring nosebleeds may warrant evaluation by a specialist.
- Identification of systemic illness may require referral to the appropriate specialist.

SIGNS TO WATCH

Persistence or recurrence of nosebleed.

PREVENTION

- Vaporizers, humidifiers, or saline sprays prevent drying of the nasal mucosa.
- Petroleum jelly applied to the nasal septum aids healing of inflamed nasal tissue.
- Reduce allergic symptoms.
- Fingernails should be cut short, and nose-picking behavior should be discouraged.
- Protective athletic equipment should be worn.

 Common Questions and Answers

Q: How should the patient with nosebleeds be positioned?
A: When possible, patients with nosebleeds should be kept upright. Those lying down may appear to have less bleeding, but this is caused by redirection of blood flow to the throat.

Obesity

 Basics

DESCRIPTION

Obesity is an excess of body fat.

SIGNS AND SYMPTOMS

A weight more than 120% of ideal body weight

CAUSES

- Multifactorial:
  - ▸ Genetic predisposition
  - ▸ Excessive caloric intake
  - ▸ Decreased physical activity
  - ▸ Decreased resting metabolic rate

SCOPE

- 25% of pediatric population is obese.
- Strong genetic predisposition:
  - ▸ One obese parent: 40% chance of having an obese child
  - ▸ Two obese parents: 70–80% chance of having an obese child

 Diagnosis

QUESTIONS THE DOCTOR MAY ASK

- Growth and weight history?
- Mental function?
- Emotional/psychological status?
- Eating behavior?
- Physical activity?
- Family characteristics?
- Parental attitude toward weight problem?
- Social relationships?
- Dietary intake?

WHAT THE DOCTOR LOOKS FOR

- Physical examination
- Thyroid enlargement
- Hypertension
- Fat distribution
- Mental development
- Sexual development

TESTS AND PROCEDURES

- Blood tests
- Bone age X-ray
- Body composition tests

 Treatment

GENERAL MEASURES

- Emphasis on lifelong behavioral changes and follow-up
- Behavior modification

ACTIVITY

The child should be encouraged to perform physical activities. Activities should be enjoyable and can involve the family.

DIET

- Reduction in total caloric intake with emphasis on decreasing fat intake
- Diet should provide sufficient calories, vitamins, minerals, and protein to promote growth.
- Diet should be individualized.

Medications

COMMONLY PRESCRIBED DRUGS

N/A

 Follow-Up

WHAT TO EXPECT

- Prognosis is poor.
- 2–5% long-term success rate (for all types of treatment)
- Best results occur with:
  ▸ Parental participation
  ▸ Treatment as a chronic disease with long-term follow-up
  ▸ Diet restriction combined with physical activity
  ▸ Realistic goals for weight loss and maintenance

 Common Questions and Answers

Q: Is childhood obesity caused by a glandular problem?
A: No, only a small percentage of obesity is caused by metabolic problems. Children with hypothyroidism are heavier and shorter than normal children.

Q: What is the most effective treatment for childhood obesity?
A: Although the long-term success of obesity therapy is less than 5% (95% regain almost all their original weight), a multidisciplinary approach consisting of behavioral modification, dietary counseling, and physical activity is the most effective. Parental participation in the therapeutic program is also important for the long-term treatment of childhood obesity.

Q: What are the causes of pediatric obesity?
A: The causes of pediatric obesity are multifactorial. They include genetic predisposition, excessive caloric intake, decreased physical activity, and decreased resting metabolic rate.

Q: What are the adverse effects of childhood obesity?
A: Psychosocial trauma is the most prevalent and devastating of the consequences. Most of the medical consequences take years to manifest. The medical problems include high blood lipids, diabetes mellitus, hypertension, cardiovascular disease, asthma, orthopedic problems, and gallbladder disease.

Parvovirus B19 Infection

 ## Basics

DESCRIPTION

Human parvovirus B19 is a common viral infection of school-aged children. Most commonly, it causes only a rash. However, it can also cause Fifth disease or erythema infectiosum, which occurs in up to 35% of school-aged children. Fifth disease can lead to arthritis and joint pain, and in some persons can cause aplastic anemia. In a pregnant woman, there is a risk that the virus can cross the placenta and infect the fetus.

SIGNS AND SYMPTOMS

- Rash on the face ("slapped cheek appearance") followed 1–4 days later by a second stage rash on the trunk and limbs
- Itching and mild joint pain
- Headache, sore throat, runny nose, joint and muscle ache, and gastrointestinal disturbances are more frequent and severe in adults.
- In children, joint symptoms are less common.
- Causes hemolytic anemia in patients with sickle cell disease

CAUSES

Infection with parvovirus B19

SCOPE

- Most parvovirus B19 infections occur in school-aged children.
- 15–35% of children 5–18 years of age have been exposed to the virus.
- Attack rates range from 15–60% of susceptible individuals.

 ## Diagnosis

QUESTIONS THE DOCTOR MAY ASK

- Fever?
- Rash?
- Joint pain?
- Medication?
- Exposure to pregnant women?

WHAT THE DOCTOR LOOKS FOR

- Approximately 20% of children and adults have no symptoms.
- Erythema infectiosum is the most common form of infection recognized.
- Anemia

TESTS AND PROCEDURES

- Blood tests
- Polymerase chain reaction (PCR)

GENERAL MEASURES

There is no specific therapy for this infection other than supportive care.

ACTIVITY

N/A

DIET

N/A

Medications

COMMONLY PRESCRIBED DRUGS

Intravenous immunoglobulin

 ## Follow-Up

WHAT TO EXPECT

- The prognosis is good for all manifestations of B19 infections. In general, these infections require supportive care only until spontaneous recovery.
- The rash of erythema infectiosum in the child or adult may last up to 20 days. It may, at times, fade and/or intensify depending on sunlight exposure, exercise, or body surface temperature changes (bathing).

SIGNS TO WATCH

Anemia

PREVENTION

N/A

 ## Common Questions and Answers

Q: When may children with B19 infection return to school?
A: Children are not infectious when the rash appears. Therefore, they may return to school or day care. The infectious period is only during the prodromal (preliminary) phase of illness, which is often unrecognized.

Pink Eye

 Basics

DESCRIPTION

Pink eye, or conjunctivitis, is an inflammation (usually infectious) involving the mucous membrane of the eye (conjunctiva).

SIGNS AND SYMPTOMS

- Redness and swelling of the eye
- Discharge from eye
- Crusting of eye, particularly in morning

CAUSE

Bacterial, viral, allergic, or toxic activation of the inflammatory response

SCOPE

- Viral conjunctivitis is extremely common and highly contagious.
- Contagious conjunctivitis may also be caused by bacteria.
- Neonatal conjunctivitis remains a significant cause of blindness worldwide.

 Diagnosis

QUESTIONS THE DOCTOR MAY ASK

N/A

WHAT THE DOCTOR LOOKS FOR

Characteristic signs and symptoms of pink eye

TESTS AND PROCEDURES

Analysis of discharge

Treatment

GENERAL MEASURES

- Usually self-limiting
- Observation
- Cool compresses may help symptoms.
- Antibiotic may be prescribed.

ACTIVITY

N/A

DIET

N/A

 ## MEDICATIONS

COMMONLY PRESCRIBED DRUGS

Antibiotics

 ## Follow-Up

WHAT TO EXPECT

- Usually self-limiting
- Visual loss or other lasting effects are rare.

 ## Common Questions and Answers

Q: Is conjunctivitis contagious?
A: All infectious conjunctivitis is contagious, but to varying degrees. Careful handling of secretions, tissues, towels, bed linens, and strict hand washing usually prevents spread. Wipe surfaces with isopropyl alcohol or dilute bleach to prevent recontamination.

Pinworms

 ## Basics

DESCRIPTION

Pinworms (*Enterobius vermicularis*) are parasites that invade the gastrointestinal tract. They cause anal itching that is usually worse at night.

SIGNS AND SYMPTOMS

- Anal itching
- Perineal itching
- Vulvovaginitis
- Bed-wetting
- Abdominal pain
- Insomnia
- Rarely occur during day

CAUSES

The intestinal parasite *E. vermicularis*

SCOPE

- Pinworms affect approximately 20% of children 5–10 years of age
- Spread by hand-to-mouth transmission
- Unrelated to personal hygiene
- Close contact is required for transmission.
- Late fall and winter infection most common
- Females are more commonly infected.

 ## Diagnosis

QUESTIONS THE DOCTOR MAY ASK

- Time of day when itching is worse?
- Exposure to illness?
- Vaginal discharge?

WHAT THE DOCTOR LOOKS FOR

- Nocturnal or early morning anal itching
- Small, white worms in the anal area or stool

TESTS AND PROCEDURES

"Scotch-tape" slide test: Parents press sticky side of clear tape to the perianal area in the morning before child rises; tape is applied to a microscope slide and examined for pinworm eggs; may need to be repeated several times

Treatment

GENERAL MEASURES

Drug therapy

ACTIVITY

N/A

DIET

N/A

 ## Medications

COMMONLY PRESCRIBED DRUGS

- Mebendazole (Vermox)
- Pyrantel pamoate
- Piperazine citrate

 ## Follow-Up

WHAT TO EXPECT

- Symptoms should improve in several days.
- Prognosis is excellent.
- Pinworms often recur.

SIGNS TO WATCH

- Recurrence
- Vaginitis

PREVENTION

- Treat all affected family members.
- Decontamination of the environment (wash sheets, towels, clothing; vacuum household)

 ## Common Questions and Answers

Q: Is this caused by poor hygiene?
A: No.

Q: Is infection with pinworms usually associated with other parasitic infections?
A: No.

Q: Can they be spread at day care?
A: Yes.

Pneumonia, Bacterial

 Basics

DESCRIPTION

Bacterial pneumonia is an acute inflammation and infection of the lung.

SIGNS AND SYMPTOMS

- Cough and fever
- Chest pain
- Headache
- Chill, with sudden onset
- Dark, thick, or rusty (bloody) sputum
- Rapid (or slow) heart rate
- Rapid breathing rate
- Shortness of breath
- Flared nostrils
- Bluish discoloration around eyes, lips, and nail beds
- Changes in the level of consciousness
- Anxiety, confusion, restlessness
- Abdominal pain
- Loss of appetite
- Profuse sweating
- Muscle aches
- Pinpoint bruises
- Nausea, vomiting, diarrhea, abdominal pain

CAUSES

Bacterial infection, spread by air or blood

SCOPE

- Children less than 2 years of age more susceptible than older children
- Twice as common in males than females
- May follow epidemics of viral infections
- All seasons; winter and spring most common

 Diagnosis

QUESTIONS THE DOCTOR MAY ASK

- Contacts with sick people?
- Previous episodes of pneumonia?
- Cough?
- Fever?
- Sputum production?
- Chest pain?
- Difficulty breathing?

WHAT THE DOCTOR LOOKS FOR

- Respirator rate
- Chest exam for abnormal signs
- Flaring of nostrils
- Movement of air into lungs
- Wheezing

TESTS AND PROCEDURES

- Blood tests
- Blood culture
- Pulse oximetry
- Arterial blood gasses
- Sampling of fluid from lungs
- Chest X-ray

 Treatment

GENERAL MEASURES

- Hospitalization may be needed.
- Antibiotic therapy

ACTIVITY

N/A

DIET

N/A

Medications

COMMONLY PRESCRIBED DRUGS

- Antibiotics
- Cefotaxime
- Erythronycin

 ## Follow-Up

WHAT TO EXPECT

- Improvement within 1 to 5 days in cases without complications
- Prognosis is excellent; less than 1% death rate in uncomplicated cases
- Longer recovery but still good outcome in other cases

SIGNS TO WATCH

- Increasing breathing difficulty
- Dehydration
- Shock
- Persistent fever

PREVENTION

Preventive antibiotics and vaccinations for children at greater risk of bacterial pneumonia

❓ Common Questions and Answers

Q: When to admit?
A: Dehydration, hypoxia, significant respiratory distress, failure of outpatient management (worsening or no response in 24-72 hours), very young age (<6 months), concern for compliance with treatment, secondary complications (effusions, empyema, pneumothorax, etc.).

Q: Who should get a follow-up chest radiograph?
A: Any child with recurrent pneumonias, persistant symptoms, severe atelectasis, unusually located infiltrates, pneumothorax, or large effusions.

Pseudotumor Cerebri

 Basics

DESCRIPTION

Pseudotumor cerebri is a condition marked by increased pressure within the skull, which may lead to visual loss or other conditions.

SIGNS AND SYMPTOMS

- Headache
- Blurred vision, double vision, other vision disturbances
- Dizziness
- Infants and young children may present with irritability, sleepiness, or incoordination.

CAUSES

- Unknown
- Associated with endocrine diseases, lead poisoning, and tetracycline

SCOPE

- The incidence in children is unknown.
- Unlike adults, male and female children are affected equally.
- Pseudotumor has been reported as early as 4 months of age, with a median age of 9 years.

 Diagnosis

QUESTIONS THE DOCTOR MAY ASK

- Headache?
- Blurred vision?
- Irritability?
- Medication?
- Lead exposure?
- Tetracyclines?

WHAT THE DOCTOR LOOKS FOR

- Optic nerve in eye exam
- Inability to gaze in lateral direction

TESTS AND PROCEDURES

- Computed tomography (CT), magnetic resonance imaging (MRI)
- Lumbar puncture (spinal tap)
- Visual testing
- Blood tests

Treatment

GENERAL MEASURES

- Removal of possible causative agents
- Treatment of associated conditions (obesity, anemia, thyroid disease)
- Surgery may be necessary when vision is impaired.

ACTIVITY

N/A

DIET

N/A

 ## Medications

COMMONLY PRESCRIBED DRUGS

- Acetazolamide (Diamox)
- Prednisone

 ## Follow-Up

WHAT TO EXPECT

- Patients should have vision tests at least monthly for 3 to 6 months.
- More frequent follow-up is required for any signs of progressive visual loss.

SIGNS TO WATCH

- Progressive visual loss
- Worsening of symptoms

PREVENTION

N/A

 ## Common Questions and Answers

Q: What are the side effects of acetazolamide?
A: Side effects of acetazolamide include GI upset, parasthesias, loss of appetite, drowsiness, metabolic acidosis, and renal stones. An alternative is furosemide.

Q: If pseudotumor occurs on tetracycline, can the child take penicillin?
A: Penicillins/cephalosporin have not been reported as a significant cause of pseudotumor.

Q: Are there any limitations on physical activity?
A: Activity can be graded entirely according to the child's symptoms.

Puberty and Pubertal Delay

Basics

DESCRIPTION

Pubertal delay is the development of puberty far later in life than average.

SIGNS AND SYMPTOMS

Delay of growth of pubic hair, breast development, and other secondary sex characteristics

CAUSE

- Most cases are constitutional or physiologic
- Infection of brain
- Trauma
- Brain tumors
- Congenital problem
- Anorexia
- Chemotherphy
- Radiation

SCOPE

Pubertal delay affects 2.5% of adolescents of both sexes.

Diagnosis

QUESTIONS THE DOCTOR MAY ASK

- Long-term growth record?
- Progression of secondary sex characteristics?
- Family history of pubertal development?
- History of drug use?

WHAT THE DOCTOR LOOKS FOR

- Physical examination
- Thyroid exam
- Neurologic and eye examination
- Breast exam
- Pubic hair
- Testicular exam

TESTS AND PROCEDURES

- Blood tests
- Urinalysis
- Genetic tests
- Bone age X-ray
- Pelvic ultrasound
- Computerized tomography (CT) and magnetic resonance imaging (MRI)
- Skull X-ray

Treatment

GENERAL MEASURES

Most patients with pubertal delay do not require drugs, but all need psychological and social support.

ACTIVITY

N/A

DIET

N/A

 ## Medications

COMMONLY PRESCRIBED DRUGS

- Most cases require no medication
- Males:
  ▶ Human chorionic gonadotropin (HCG)
  ▶ Testosterone
  ▶ Gonadotropin releasing hormone (GnRh) or gonadotropin
- Females:
  ▶ Ethinyl estradiol
  ▶ Oral estrogens
  ▶ Medroxyprogesterone acetate (Provera)
  ▶ Combined oral contraceptive

 ## Follow-Up

WHAT TO EXPECT

- Outcome depends on cause of pubertal delay.
- Hormone replacement therapy may be life-long.

SIGNS TO WATCH

- Endocrine problems
- Development of puberty
- Neurologic problems

PREVENTION

N/A

 ## Common Questions and Answers

Q: Since approximately 95% of pubertal delay is constitutional or physiologic in nature, when can I avoid an expensive work-up and just observe the patient?

A: Unfortunately, only the spontaneous onset of puberty after time confirms the diagnosis of constitutional delay. To make a presumptive diagnosis of constitutional delay, pathology must be ruled out. Physical examination, including genital anatomy and smell sense, must be normal, with no signs or symptoms consistent with chronic disease. The history, including nutritional history and review of systems, must be negative. The screening blood work must be negative. Although not always indicated, the next level of tests can be ordered. Growth must be progressing at least 3.7 cm per year and bone age must be delayed 1.5 to 4.0 years compared to chronological age. Normal prepubertal levels of LH and FSH must be present. Presumptive diagnosis is strongly supported, but not proven, by a positive family history and a height between the 3rd and 25th percentile.

Rash

Basics

DESCRIPTION

Also called urticaria or hives, a rash consists of a single or multiple itchy raised bumps on the skin, typically pale with a red halo. A rash may subside rapidly, resulting in no scars or change in pigmentation. A rash may recur.

- Acute rash:
  - ► Reaction to many stimuli
  - ► May be unusual response to drug exposure
  - ► Subsides over several hours
- Chronic rash:
  - ► Persists more than 6 weeks in 30% of cases
  - ► Cold rash: from cooling and rewarming. Can be fatal. This form may affect several members of a family with fever, chills, joint and muscle pain, and headache.
- Heat rash: small (5–10 mm) spots on upper trunk from overheating, hot shower
- Exercise-induced rash: from extreme exercise; marked by swelling, wheezing, low blood pressure.
- Solar rash: result of exposure to sunlight. Onset in minutes; subsides in 1 to 2 hours.

SIGNS AND SYMPTOMS

- Rash may appear alone or with swelling.
- May occur with generalized allergic reaction; potentially fatal
- Single or multiple raised, pale spots surrounded by a red halo
- Intensely itchy
- May occur anywhere on body
- Spots are variably sized
- Acute rash develops rapidly, resolves spontaneously in less than 48 hours.

CAUSES

- Allergy-triggering substance may be inhaled, eaten, or contacted on the skin.
- Drug reaction
- Food or food additive allergy
- Insect bite, sting
- Infection
- Physical trauma (heat, cold, sunlight)

SCOPE

Rash affects about 1 in 1000 persons, or 15–20% of the United States population at some time during life.

Diagnosis

QUESTIONS THE DOCTOR MAY ASK

N/A

WHAT THE DOCTOR LOOKS FOR

- Previous history of rash
- Known exposures and ingestions
- Underlying medical problems
- For chronic rash: symptom diary including activity, diet, illnesses, sun exposure, and medications
- Physical examination

TESTS AND PROCEDURES

- Urinalysis
- Blood tests may be done to identify signs of infection or inflammation.
- A sample of skin tissue obtained by biopsy may be examined microscopically.
- Tests may be done to evaluate allergies to foods or other substances.
- Special tests include:
  - ▶ Cold rash: ice cube test (ice cube placed on skin 5 minutes, observed 10–15 minutes)
  - ▶ Exercise-induced rash: exercise challenge; methacholine skin test
  - ▶ Solar rash: expose to defined wavelengths of light
  - ▶ Delayed-pressure rash: apply 5–10-pound sandbag for 3 hours, observe
  - ▶ Water rash: apply tap water at different temperatures
  - ▶ Vibratory rash: apply vibration 4–5 minutes with a lab mixing device, observe

 Treatment

GENERAL MEASURES

- Acute cases don't usually require a full work-up.
- Cool, moist compresses help control itching.
- Avoid substances that provoke allergies if they are known. Use antihistamines if accidentally re-exposed.

ACTIVITY

As desired. Avoid overheating.

DIET

As desired. Avoid foods suspected as possible allergy triggers.

 Medications

COMMONLY PRESCRIBED DRUGS

- Antihistamines
- Corticosteroids
- Epinephrine

 Follow-Up

WHAT TO EXPECT

- Prognosis is good.
- Acute rash: improvement within 30 minutes of antihistamine administration; almost immediately with epinephrine
- Chronic rash: may persist intermittently for weeks to years

SIGNS TO WATCH

Airway compromise, wheezing, hoarse voice, difficulty breathing or swallowing

PREVENTION

- Sun screens, protective clothing, or sun avoidance for solar rash
- Avoid causative agents (foods, contacts, inhalants, medications).

 Common Questions and Answers

Q: Should patients with chronic rash be referred to a specialist?
A: If rash persists for greater than 6 weeks and no underlying cause is identified, the patient should be referred to an allergist or immunologist for evaluation and treatment because it may be a sign of underlying systemic disease.

Respiratory Syncytial Virus

 ## Basics

DESCRIPTION

Respiratory syncytial virus (RSV) is a common cause of lower respiratory system infection of children.

SIGNS AND SYMPTOMS

- Nasal discharge
- Cough
- Fever
- Rapid breathing
- Difficulty breathing
- Episodes of apnea or a bluish discoloration around lips, eyes, and nail beds (cyanosis)
- Lethargy
- Dehydration
- Ear infection

CAUSES

Respiratory syncytial virus

SCOPE

- Peak incidence: first 2 years of life
- 50% of children affected by their first birthday
- 40–70% of preschool children and 20% of school-age children are reinfected.

 ## Diagnosis

QUESTIONS THE DOCTOR MAY ASK

- Did the child stop breathing?
- Nasal discharge?
- Fever?
- Cough?
- Rapid breathing?
- Fluid intake?

WHAT THE DOCTOR LOOKS FOR

- Nasal discharge
- Ear infection
- Red throat
- Red eyes
- Rapid breath
- Grunting
- Wheezing
- Fatigue

TESTS AND PROCEDURES

- Blood tests
- Swab of nose or throat for microbiological analysis
- Pulse oximetry

 ## Treatment

GENERAL MEASURES

- Supportive care
- Monitoring
- Oxygen and/or breathing assistance may be needed.
- Fluids

ACTIVITY

N/A

DIET

Encourage adequate fluids and nutrition.

Medications

COMMONLY PRESCRIBED DRUGS

- Ribavirin–used in hospitalized patients
- Corticosteroids
- Aminophylline and ventolin not proven to be effective

 ## Follow-Up

WHAT TO EXPECT

- Fever usually improves over 48 hours.
- Respiratory symptoms improve on the second to fifth day of illness.
- Child may wheeze for a period of time after illness.
- Most infants with mild to moderate disease recover well.
- Some children have more severe disease requiring hospitalization.
- Children with underlying disease are at greater risk.
- Reinfection can occur throughout life.

SIGNS TO WATCH

- Breathing rate greater than 60 breaths per minute or signs of respiratory failure (cyanosis)
- Lethargy, altered level of consciousness
- Prolonged high fever

PREVENTION

Good hand-washing practices can help reduce spread of infection.

 ## Common Questions and Answers

Q: For how long is my child contagious?
A: Children are contagious from 24 hours before the development of symptoms until 21 days after the onset of symptoms.

Q: Will my child develop asthma because of the wheezing that is occurring now?
A: Airway reactivity may continue for months or even years in some children. It is impossible to predict future episodes of asthma, but the child should be monitored over time.

Rhinitis, Allergic

 Basics

DESCRIPTION

Allergic rhinitis, or hay fever, is a reaction to airborne allergens. The condition may be seasonal or perennial depending on climate and individual response. Seasonal responses are usually to grasses, trees, and weeds. Perennial responses may be caused by house-dust mites, mold antigens, and animal body products (dander).

SIGNS AND SYMPTOMS

- Nasal stuffiness and congestion
- Sneezing, often in spasms
- Watery eyes
- Dark circles under eyes, "allergic shiners"
- Long eye lashes
- Sensation of plugged ears
- Sleeping difficulties
- Fatigue
- Mouth breathing
- Scratchy throat
- Voice change
- Irritating cough
- Postnasal drip
- Loss or alteration of smell
- Itchy nose, eyes, ears, and palate

CAUSES

- Animal proteins: molds, house-dust mites, danders, dried saliva, and urine
- Insect debris: cockroaches, locusts, fish food
- Other indoor allergens, such as cigarette smoke, hair spray, paint
- Pollen (tree pollens in early spring, grass in late spring and early summer, ragweed in late summer and autumn)
- Multiple environmental factors
- Changes in air temperature

SCOPE

- Affects 8–20% of children and 15–30% of adolescents.
- It is estimated that up to 75% of children with asthma also have allergic rhinitis.
- Most commonly begins during childhood and young adulthood

 Diagnosis

QUESTIONS THE DOCTOR MAY ASK

- Eye redness and itching?
- Are the symptoms seasonal, perennial, or episodic?
- What makes symptoms worse: pollen, animals, cigarette smoke, dust, molds?
- History of fever?
- Family history of allergies?

WHAT THE DOCTOR LOOKS FOR

- Stuffy nose, sneezing, itching, and runny nose
- Noisy breathing, snoring, cough, and repeated throat clearing
- Sensation of plugged ears and wheezing
- Physical examination
- Nasal redness or paleness
- Dark circles under eye

TESTS AND PROCEDURES

- Blood tests
- Analysis of nasal discharge
- Sweat test if cystic fibrosis suspected or if nasal polyps are present
- Hearing tests
- Allergy testing
- The nose may be examined by rhinoscopy.
- X-rays of sinuses or chest

Treatment

GENERAL MEASURES

- Therapy should begin with identification and elimination of known/suspected allergens.
- Steam inhalation
- Saline drops
- Immunotherapy
- Surgery may be recommended.

ACTIVITY

N/A

DIET

N/A

 ## Medications

COMMONLY PRESCRIBED DRUGS

- Guaifenesin–decreases mucus
- Diphenhydramine (Benadryl)
- Astemizole (Hismanal), terfenadine (Seldane)
- Cromolyn (Nasalcrom)
- Oral decongestants: ephedrine, pseudoephedrine, phenylephrine, or phenylpropanolamine
- Topical decongestants: phenylephrine (NeoSynephrine), and oxymetazoline (Afrin)
- Combined oral decongestants and antihistamines: chlorpheniramine, methscopolamine, phenylephrine (Extendryl) and chlorpheniramine and pseudoephedrine (Atrohist)
- Topical steroids: beclomethasone (Vancenase, Beconase), flunisolide (Nasalide), fluticasone propionate (Flonase), triamcinolone (Nasacort)

 ## Follow-Up

WHAT TO EXPECT

- Improvement within days to weeks
- Prognosis is generally good, when environmental factors are eliminated and when medical therapy is used appropriately.
- Complete recovery occurs in 5 to 10% of patients.

SIGNS TO WATCH

Fever, prolonged or severe headache, dizziness, pain, or pus discharge

PREVENTION

- Minimize exposure to dust mites and other allergens (e.g., avoid dander).
- Remove carpets if individual is markedly sensitive to dust mites.
- Solutions containing tannic acid eliminate animal allergens.
- Solutions containing benzyl benzoate kill mites.

 ## Common Questions and Answers

Q: How does one minimize exposure to dust mites?
A: Keep household temperature low; maintain humidity at approximately 40–50%; wash linens at hot temperatures, weekly; use a microfilter when vacuuming; place mattress and boxspring in airtight plastic casing; use air conditioning; use high-efficiency particulate air filter units.

Rickets

 Basics

DESCRIPTION

Rickets is the undermineralization of growing bones, causing them to soften and bend.

SIGNS AND SYMPTOMS

- Alterations in the long bones
- Widening of wrists and knees
- Bowed legs
- Muscle weakness
- Awkward gait
- Bone pain
- Delayed standing, walking
- Pathologic fractures
- Loss of appetite
- Seizures
- Slowed growth (short stature)
- Deformity of the head
- Dental cavities

CAUSES

- Calcium deficiency
- Vitamin D deficiency
- Phosphorus deficiency

SCOPE

- Children at high risk for rickets:
  - ▶ Small, premature infants
  - ▶ Breast-fed infants who are not exposed to the sun and who do not receive supplemental vitamin D
  - ▶ Children with chronic kidney disease
  - ▶ Children with biliary atresia or chronic liver disease
  - ▶ Children with inflammatory bowel disease

 Diagnosis

QUESTIONS THE DOCTOR MAY ASK

- Family history of rickets?
- Vitamin D intake?
- Exposure to sun?
- Calcium intake?
- Diarrhea?
- Growth records?
- Prematurity?

WHAT THE DOCTOR LOOKS FOR

- Length and weight
- Enlargement of front of head
- Large liver
- Tender extremities
- Bowed legs
- Swelling of ribs
- Irritability

TESTS AND PROCEDURES

- Blood tests
- Urinalysis
- X-rays of knee and wrist
- Dual energy X-ray absorptiometry

 Treatment

GENERAL MEASURES

- Diet
- Calcium
- Vitamin D
- Exposure to sun

ACTIVITY

N/A

DIET

If infant, formula may be adjusted

Medications

COMMONLY PRESCRIBED DRUGS

- Calcium
- Vitamin D
- Calcitrol
- Phosphorus

 ## Follow-Up

WHAT TO EXPECT

- Frequent monitoring (every 2–3 months) should be done when vitamin D therapy is used.
- Improvement should be seen within 6 weeks.

SIGNS TO WATCH

- Growth
- Bone swelling
- Gait
- Bowed legs

PREVENTION

N/A

 ## Common Questions and Answers

Q: Why are premature infants prone to rickets?
A: Premature infants have higher calcium and phosphorus requirements than full-term infants. They also tend to be sicker at birth and sometimes have feeding difficulties or malabsorption.

Q: What are the effects of rickets?
A: The most common medical effects of rickets include pathologic bone fractures, slowed growth (short stature), and muscle weakness.

Q: Can rickets be treated effectively?
A: Yes, rickets can be treated effectively with the right amount and right combination of calcium, phosphorus, or vitamin D supplementation.

Rocky Mountain Spotted Fever

 Basics

DESCRIPTION

Rocky Mountain spotted fever (RMSF), an acute, potentially fatal illness transmitted by tick bite, is marked by headache, fever, and rash.

SIGNS AND SYMPTOMS

- Fever
- Rash
- Headache
- Nausea, vomiting
- Abdominal pain
- Muscle and joint pain
- Enlarged lymph nodes
- Cough
- Central nervous system dysfunction (stupor, confusion, coma)

CAUSES

RMSF is caused by the bacterium *Rickettsia rickettsii*, which is transmitted by the bite of ticks.

SCOPE

- April to September most common
- Corresponds to period of greatest tick and outdoor activity
- Endemic to South Atlantic and West-South-Central regions
- Less often seen in Rocky Mountain states
- Also found in Mexico and Central and South America
- Two-thirds of patients are younger than 15 years of age (especially 5–9 years of age).

 Diagnosis

QUESTIONS THE DOCTOR MAY ASK

- Abrupt or gradual onset of fever, headache, rash, confusion, muscle ache, nausea, vomiting, abdominal pain?
- Tick bite history in only 50–70% of cases

WHAT THE DOCTOR LOOKS FOR

- Central nervous system disorders
- Rash on palm
- Irregular heartbeat
- Eye exam
- Evaluation of abdominal pain

TESTS AND PROCEDURES

- Blood tests
- Chest X-ray
- Arterial blood gasses
- Electrocardiogram (EKG)
- Echocardiogram
- Identification of bacteria

 Treatment

GENERAL MEASURES

- Supportive care is very important.
- Fluid, salt replacement as indicated
- Blood transfusion may be needed.
- Antibiotics

ACTIVITY

N/A

DIET

N/A

Medications

COMMONLY PRESCRIBED DRUGS

- Tetracycline
- Doxycycline
- Chloramphenicol
- Corticosteroids
- Vitamin K
- Albumin

 ## Follow-Up

WHAT TO EXPECT

- Recovery the rule if treated in first week
- Majority improve if treated early.
- Expect improvement in 24 to 36 hours and break of fever in 2 to 3 days.
- Death rate is approximately 3–7%.

SIGNS TO WATCH

- Neurologic problem
- Cough
- Electrolyte problem

PREVENTION

- Avoid tick-infested areas and tick contact. Tuck pant legs into boots, limit skin access to ticks, inspect skin frequently.
- Use tick repellants.
- Remove ticks early because ticks must attach and feed for 4 to 6 or more hours to transmit disease. Avoid direct contact with tick during removal. Remove tick with tweezers at point of attachment and clean wound.
- Immunity conferred after disease

 ## Common Questions and Answers

Q: Should a child with a tick bite receive antibiotic preventive when a tick is discovered?
A: To contract disease, one must be bitten by a tick that actually carries the disease (low risk), the tick must transmit the Rickettsia before it is removed (low risk), and the Rickettsia must be the cause of disease (low risk). There is no evidence that preventive therapy is necessary or effective in preventing disease. If considered, one must weigh risks and benefits of the therapy to be used.

Roseola

 Basics

DESCRIPTION

Roseola infantum is a common illness in preschool-aged children. It is characterized by fever lasting 3–7 days followed by rapid improvement and the appearance of a blanching rash (usually on the fourth day of illness) lasting only 1–2 days. In a small number of cases, the illness can lead to seizures or other lingering effects.

SIGNS AND SYMPTOMS

- Fever for period of 3 to 5 days, commonly in the range of 102–105°F (38.9–40.6°C)
- Rash appears as the fever disappears and lasts for 1 to 2 days.
- Mild cough and runny nose

CAUSES

Viral infection–adenovirus, parovirus, human herpes virus-6

SCOPE

- Roseola can occur throughout the year; outbreaks have occurred in all seasons of the year.
- Roseola affects children from 3 months to 4 years of age; the peak age is 7–13 months.
- 90% of cases occur in the first 2 years of life.
- Cases occur in males and females equally.
- Incubation period is 5–15 days.

 Diagnosis

QUESTIONS THE DOCTOR MAY ASK

- Fever?
- Onset of rash?
- Exposure to ill people?
- Seizure?

WHAT THE DOCTOR LOOKS FOR

- Rash appears after fever ebbs
- Seizure
- Purpura, small hemorrhage in skin

TESTS AND PROCEDURES

Blood tests

 Treatment

GENERAL MEASURES

Supportive care

ACTIVITY

N/A

DIET

N/A

Follow-Up

WHAT TO EXPECT

The vast majority of children with roseola infantum recover without lasting effects.

SIGNS TO WATCH

N/A

PREVENTION

The virus associated with roseola infantum is usually transmitted via respiratory secretions or the fecal/oral spread. Hand washing may help prevent the spread of the disease.

 Common Questions and Answers

Q: When can the child with roseola return to day care?
A: As soon as the child is without fever, there is no infectious risk of spread. They may return to day care even with rash visible.

Q: Will there be long-term effects in the child who has a seizure associated with roseola?
A: In general, these seizures are typical febrile seizures that hold no risk for long-term neurologic effects, i.e., epilepsy.

Scabies

Basics

DESCRIPTION

Scabies is a contagious skin disease caused by infestation by the mite *Sarcoptes scabiei*.

SIGNS AND SYMPTOMS

- Generalized itching
- Itching during sleep hours
- Scabies burrow between fingers and into the skin of the wrists, hands, feet, penis, scrotum, buttocks, and waistline.
- Blisters and welts
- Peeling skin
- Reddening

CAUSES

Skin infestation by the mite *S. scabiei*

SCOPE

- Affects all age groups
- Epidemics are reported to occur in a 15-year cycle.
- Close personal contact with an infested human is required for transmission.
- Mite can live isolated from a human body for 2 to 3 days.

Diagnosis

QUESTIONS THE DOCTOR MAY ASK

- Where did the rash first appear and has the rash changed over time?
- Is the rash itchy?
- Does anyone else in the family have a similar rash?
- Changes in rash?

WHAT THE DOCTOR LOOKS FOR

- Burrows in skin, especially between fingers

TESTS AND PROCEDURES

Skin scrapings for analysis

Treatment

GENERAL MEASURES

- All family members and close contacts should be treated concurrently regardless of clinical symptoms (contacts may be infested without symptoms).
- Bedding, clothing, and items of close contact should be washed and dried in hot temperatures at the time of treatment.

ACTIVITY

N/A

DIET

N/A

Medications

COMMONLY PRESCRIBED DRUGS

- Permethrin cream (Elimite)
- Lindane
- Crotamiton cream
- Sulfur in a petrolatum base
- Topical steroids
- Antibiotics if infection also present

 ## Follow-Up

WHAT TO EXPECT

- Itching may take up to 4 weeks to resolve after effective treatment.
- Prognosis is excellent.

SIGNS TO WATCH

Persistence of symptoms

PREVENTION

N/A

 ## Common Questions and Answers

Q: How did my child get scabies?
A: From close contact with an infested person.

Q: How long will my child continue to itch?
A: Itching may continue for weeks; the use of topical hydrocortisone may be helpful.

Q: Do I need to wash my child's bedding in a special detergent?
A: Simply wash all bedding in hot soapy water after your child has been treated.

Seizures

 ## Basics

DESCRIPTION

Seizures are a transient involuntary alteration of consciousness, behavior, movement, or sensation caused by neurologic disturbances. Epilepsy is one type of seizure disorder. Status epilepticus is defined as 30 minutes or more of seizure activity, or two or more seizures within 30 minutes without a full recovery of consciousness between seizures. Seizures are classified as partial (beginning in one part of the brain) or generalized (beginning in both sides of the brain).

SIGNS AND SYMPTOMS

- Fever (if caused by infection)
- Changes in level of consciousness
- Involuntary muscular contraction

CAUSES

- Brain tumor
- Brain injury
- Stroke
- Poisoning
- Fever
- Drugs
- Abnormal blood vessels
- Metabolic diseases

SCOPE

4–6% of children have at least one seizure in the first 16 years of life; the highest incidence is in childhood, with 30% of first seizures occurring before age 4 years and nearly 80% occurring before age 20 years.

 ## Diagnosis

QUESTIONS THE DOCTOR MAY ASK

- Fever?
- Head Trauma?
- Medication?
- Birth history?
- Headache?
- Change in vision?
- Change in behavior?
- Change in gait or balance?
- History of seizures or neurologic abnormality?

WHAT THE DOCTOR LOOKS FOR

- Physical examination
- Evidence of trauma to the head
- Eye exam
- Coordination
- Reflexes
- Muscle weakness
- Gait
- Balance
- Mental status

TESTS AND PROCEDURES

- Blood tests
- Urinalysis
- Pulse oximetry
- Lumbar puncture (spinal tap)
- Electroencephalogram (EEG)
- Computed tomography (CT) or magnetic resonance imaging (MRI)

 ## Treatment

GENERAL MEASURES

- Protect the child having a seizure from hurting self; cushion head.
- Keep airway open.
- Most seizures are self-limiting.
- Do not put fingers or other items in person's mouth during seizure.
- Medication to control seizures

ACTIVITY

Few restrictions need to be placed on patients with epilepsy, with the exceptions of driving or operating heavy machinery in adolescents, or particularly dangerous sports, such as scuba diving, parachuting, and rock climbing.

DIET

N/A

Medications

COMMONLY PRESCRIBED DRUGS

- Carbamazepine, phenytoin, valproate, phenobarbital
- Ethosuximide

Follow-Up

WHAT TO EXPECT

- Most seizures are self-limiting.
- No convincing evidence exists that an isolated brief seizure causes brain damage.
- Serious injury from a brief seizure is rare and usually is related to loss of consciousness and falls.
- The reported risk of recurrence after a single unprovoked seizure in children varies from 27 to 40%.

SIGNS TO WATCH

- Progressive number of seizures
- Change in behavior

PREVENTION

N/A

Common Questions and Answers

Q: How do you know my child has epilepsy?
A: The term epilepsy is applied to children with recurrent (greater than 1) seizure not caused by fever or other transient disturbance, because in general these children have a high (greater than 60%) probability of further recurrences.

Q: Will my child always be an epileptic?
A: Depending on the circumstances, children may "grow out" of their seizure disorder. In many cases, antiseizure drugs can be discontinued if the child has been seizure-free for 2 years.

Q: Why take an antiseizure drug?
A: The purpose of antiseizure medication is to prevent status epilepticus and to prevent accidents and interference with normal behavior associated with brief seizures.

Seizures, Febrile

 Basics

DESCRIPTION

Febrile seizures are brief (less than 15 minutes) seizures occurring during rise of fever in otherwise normal children between the ages of 6 months and 5 years of age.

SIGNS AND SYMPTOMS

- Loss of consciousness
- Uncontrollable, chaotic muscle contraction

CAUSE

Associated with a rise in body temperature, may be genetic

SCOPE

3–4% of children will experience a febrile seizure.

 Diagnosis

QUESTIONS THE DOCTOR MAY ASK

- Fever-maximum temperature?
- Headaches, vomiting, weakness?
- Change in behavior?
- History of seizures or neurologic conditions?
- Family history of seizures?

WHAT THE DOCTOR LOOKS FOR

- Physical examination
- Temperature
- Source of fever
- Head trauma
- Rash
- Uneven reflexes
- Mental status
- Motor strength

TESTS AND PROCEDURES

- Lumbar puncture (spinal tap)
- Electroencephalogram (EEG)
- Magnetic resonance imaging (MRI)

 Treatment

GENERAL MEASURES

Because only one-third of children with an initial febrile seizure have a second seizure, treatment of a single febrile seizure is not indicated.

ACTIVITY

N/A

DIET

N/A

Medications

COMMONLY PRESCRIBED DRUGS

- Diazepam
- Phenobarbital
- Valproate
- Primidone

 ## Follow-Up

WHAT TO EXPECT

- One-third of children who have a first simple febrile seizure have a second at the time of subsequent febrile illnesses, and half of these have a third febrile seizure.
- One-half of the recurrences occur within 6 months of the first febrile seizure, three-quarters within a year, and 90% within 2 years.
- Less than 9% of children with febrile seizures have more than three.
- The risk of recurrence is increased if the child has a family history of febrile seizures or if the first febrile seizure occurs before 12 months of age or at a body temperature less than 104°F.
- There is no evidence that occasional febrile seizures cause neurologic damage, mental retardation, a decrease in IQ, cerebral palsy, or learning problems.

 ## Common Questions and Answers

Q: What should be done if the child has another febrile seizure?
A: Emergency measures include lying the child down with the head turned to the side to prevent inhaling vomit or saliva; place nothing in the mouth.

Q: What restrictions should be placed on the general activity of a child with recurrent febrile seizures?
A: No specific restrictions are recommended.

Q: What is the long term outlook?
A: Most children suffer no consequences after a febrile seizure.

Q: What is a complex febrile seizure?
A: Those that last more than 15 minutes, are focal or recur within one day.

Q: My 4-month old has a fever and a seizure. Is this a febrile seizure?
A: No. Seizures in a 4 month old are potentially more serious and require a more complete evaluation.

Serum Sickness

Basics

DESCRIPTION

Serum sickness is an immune system response resulting from injection of protein or nonprotein medications.

SIGNS AND SYMPTOMS

- Fever
- Rash
- Swollen lymph nodes
- Blood in urine
- Joint pain, swelling, or warmth
- Headache

CAUSES

- Serum used for prevention and treatment of botulism, diphtheria, tetanus, gangrene, black widow spider bites, snakebites, organ transplant rejection
- Snake venoms
- Thrombolytic ("clot-dissolving") therapy
- Nonprotein drugs, including antibiotics

SCOPE

- Develops 6–10 days after exposure to offending agent.

Diagnosis

QUESTIONS THE DOCTOR MAY ASK

- Joint pain or swelling?
- Headaches?
- Abdomen pain?
- Exposure 1–14 days before symptoms, especially medications?
- Description and evolution of rash?

WHAT THE DOCTOR LOOKS FOR

- Rash
- Fever
- Swollen glands
- Warm or tender joints
- Large liver or spleen

TESTS AND PROCEDURES

- Urinalysis
- Blood tests
- Electrocardiogram (EKG)
- Stool analysis
- Computed tomography (CT) of head

Treatment

GENERAL MEASURES

- Eliminate the offending agent.
- Severe cases may require hospitalization.
- Most patients are treated as outpatients with phone and office follow-up.

ACTIVITY

N/A

DIET

N/A

Medications

COMMONLY PRESCRIBED DRUGS

- Antihistamines
- Nonsteroidal anti-inflammatory drugs (NSAIDS)
- Corticosteroids
- Epinephrine

 Follow-Up

WHAT TO EXPECT

- Usually self-limited; resolves in 2 to 3 weeks; may last longer or recur
- Overall excellent prognosis; rarely fatal

SIGNS TO WATCH

Respiratory distress, change in mental status, chest pain

PREVENTION

Avoid implicated drugs unless they are absolutely indicated.

 Common Questions and Answers

Q: Is my child now unable to receive antibiotics?
A: The offending antibiotic should never again be prescribed to the affected child. Repeat exposure most likely results in a serum sickness response again, often more quickly than the initial event. However, many antibiotics from other drug families are not associated with serum sickness.

Q: Will my child have long-lasting effects such as arthritis from this disease?
A: No, most children recover completely .

Sexual Abuse

Basics

DESCRIPTION

Sexual abuse is the involvement of a child in sexual activities that he/she cannot understand, for which he/she is not developmentally prepared, and to which he/she cannot give informed consent, and that violate societal taboos.

SIGNS AND SYMPTOMS

- Trauma to genetalia
- Sexually transmitted disease
- Withdrawn behavior

CAUSES

Complex interaction of societal, familial, and individual factors

SCOPE

- Approximately 150,000 substantiated cases are identified each year in the United States. This is likely to be a significant underestimation of the actual numbers.
- Girls are victimized more commonly than boys, who represent approximately 20% of cases reported to child protection agencies each year.
- Sexual abuse of boys is believed to be under-reported.
- Children of all ages are victimized, with peak age of vulnerability being 7–13 years for boys and girls.
- Race and socioeconomic status are not believed to play a role in the epidemiology of sexual abuse.

Diagnosis

QUESTIONS THE DOCTOR MAY ASK

- Identity of alleged perpetrator?
- Last contact?
- Previous reports of abuse?
- Change in behavior?
- Vaginal discharge?

WHAT THE DOCTOR LOOKS FOR

- Signs of sexual abuse
- Conditions associated with sexual abuse
- External genetalia
- Condition of hymen
- Vaginal discharge

TESTS AND PROCEDURES

- Blood tests
- Cultures for microbiological analysis
- Forensic evidence collection

Treatment

GENERAL MEASURES

- Ensure safety of the child.
- Suspected abuse must be reported to local child welfare agency.
- Suspected sexual abuse must be reported to law enforcement.
- Treatment of sexually transmitted disease
- Sitz baths for comfort
- Cases are investigated by child welfare and/or the police.
- Need for foster care placement and ongoing supervision is decided by investigation.
- Most children are referred for short- or long-term counseling.

ACTIVITY

N/A

DIET

N/A

Medications

COMMONLY PRESCRIBED DRUGS

- Antibiotics
- Pregnancy prevention (e.g., hormonal contraceptive) for adolescents
- Tetanus booster

 ## Follow-Up

WHAT TO EXPECT

- Minor physical injuries, such as abrasions, contusions, or minor lacerations, heal within a few days.
- More extensive injuries (e.g., deep lacerations, tears) may take weeks to months to heal.
- Resolution of the emotional impact of abuse is very slow and may take years.
- Prognosis varies greatly depending on specifics of abuse sustained and the support systems available.

SIGNS TO WATCH

- Persistent physical/genital complaints
- Aggressive, hypersexual, and/or withdrawn behavior, which may be a consequence of having been abused
- Patient victimizing a younger child. Young perpetrators are often victims of previous abuse. It is important to get help for the child perpetrator so that the pattern of abuse does not continue.

PREVENTION

The effectiveness of sexual abuse prevention programs is difficult to measure. Although children who are taught about personal safety learn from the experience, it is unknown whether behavior is changed by such education.

 ## Common Questions and Answers

Q: Are sexually transmitted diseases always transmitted sexually?
A: No. All sexually transmitted diseases may be transmitted from mother to infant. Casual transmission of sexually transmitted diseases could occur for some organisms, but not for others.

Q: How often do sexually abused children have physical evidence of the abuse?
A: In the majority of cases, there are no specific physical indicators of abuse. Only a small minority of patients have physical evidence considered diagnostic of abuse.

Sexual Ambiguity

 Basics

DESCRIPTION

Genitalia can be defined as ambiguous when it is not possible to categorize the gender of the child based on outward appearances.

SIGNS AND SYMPTOMS

- Genitalia that is not clearly male or female
- Divided scrotum
- Fusion of labia
- Abnormal position of urethra
- Atypical penis

CAUSES

- Genetic disorders
- Disorders of sex gland (gonad) development
- Other metabolic disorders
- Multiple birth defects
- Unknown

SCOPE

Disorders causing sexual ambiguity occur congenitally and are apparent during the newborn period.

 Diagnosis

QUESTIONS THE DOCTOR MAY ASK

- Pregnancy history?
- Family history?
- Infection?
- Drug ingestion?

WHAT THE DOCTOR LOOKS FOR

- Physical examination
- Placement of urethra (opening to bladder)
- Size of penis
- Scrotum
- Pressure of testicles

TESTS AND PROCEDURES

- Blood tests
- Genetic tests
- Pelvic ultrasound
- Urethrogram

Treatment

GENERAL MEASURES

- Gender assignment should be done as early as possible.
- Gender assignment is based more on genital appearance than on genetics.
- Surgery may be necessary.
- Drug treatment may be necessary.

ACTIVITY

N/A

DIET

N/A

 ## Medications

COMMONLY PRESCRIBED DRUGS

Hydrocortisone, fludrocortisone, cortisol

 ## Follow-Up

WHAT TO EXPECT

- Families should receive appropriate counseling.
- Hormone replacement therapy at puberty may be necessary.
- Long-term follow-up

SIGNS TO WATCH

N/A

PREVENTION

N/A

 ## Common Questions and Answers

Q: When genetalia are ambiguous, how do you raise the child, as male or female?
A: This is a complex problem which requires a rapid diagnosis, review of laboratory tests and then a team decision. Recent studies show sexual issues persist.

Sexual Precocity

 Basics

DESCRIPTION

Sexual precocity is defined as sexual development before age 8 in girls and age 9 in boys.

SIGNS AND SYMPTOMS

- Breast development, pubic hair growth in girls
- Pubic hair growth, changes in testicle and penis size in boys

CAUSES

- Central precocious puberty is associated with brain trauma, tumors or infection.
- Peripheral precocious puberty is associated with gonadal or adrenal problems.

SCOPE

- Precocious puberty is more common in girls.
- Precocious puberty in boys is more likely to be associated with underlying disease.

 Diagnosis

QUESTIONS THE DOCTOR MAY ASK

- Careful chronology of physical changes, growth spurt, onset of menstrual cycles
- Family history of early puberty
- Physical examination
- Exposure to hormones?

TESTS AND PROCEDURES

- Blood tests
- Measurement of testicular volume
- Bone age X-ray
- Magnetic resonance imaging (MRI) of head
- Ultrasound

Treatment

GENERAL MEASURES

Depends on cause of precocity

ACTIVITY

N/A

DIET

N/A

 ## Medications

COMMONLY PRESCRIBED DRUGS

Hormone treatment (e.g., gonadotropin releasing hormone [GnRH] agonists)

 ## Follow-Up

WHAT TO EXPECT

- Outcome depends on cause.
- Treatment of central precocious puberty usually results in cessation of menses within 2 months, slow down or cessation of pubertal changes over 4–6 months, and decreased acceleration of bone age within 1 year.
- With treatment, improvement in predicted height is achieved, but most do not reach target height predicted.

SIGNS TO WATCH

Moodiness, development of acne, or recurrence or failure to suppress menstruation

PREVENTION

N/A

 ## Common Questions and Answers

Q: If a child has some pubertal changes already, can they be reversed?
A: If GnRH agonists are used, menstruation ceases, and breast tissue and pubic hair often regress.

Sexually Transmitted Disease

 Basics

DESCRIPTION

Sexually transmitted disease (STD) is an infectious disease acquired by sexual behavior. Intercourse is not required to spread STD. Child sexual abuse must be considered in all cases of sexually transmitted disease in prepubescent children outside the neonatal period and in any nonsexually active adolescent.

- Pediatric gonococcal infections are categorized by age group: the neonatal or newborn infant, prepubertal children, and sexually active adolescents. Neonatal gonococcal diseases include eye infection, scalp abscess (complication after fetal scalp monitoring), and, rarely, vaginitis or systemic disease. Gonococcal disease in the prepubescent age group usually occurs in the genital tract with vaginitis as the most common presenting manifestation.
- Cervicitis is infection and inflammation of the cervix.
- Genital warts, also called venereal warts or condyloma acuminata, are soft, skin-colored, fleshy warts that are caused by the human papilloma virus (HPV). Warts appear in the vagina, on the cervix, around the external genitalia and rectum, and occasionally in the throat. Warts can appear singly or in groups.
- Herpes simplex is a viral disease usually causing painful blisters that often occur in clusters on skin, the eye, or mucous membranes. Newborns or those with immune system disorders are at greater risk for complications or death.
- Pelvic inflammatory disease is infection and inflammation of the upper female reproductive tract.
- Vaginal discharge may be normal in newborns or may be caused by infection and inflammation.

SIGNS AND SYMPTOMS

- Inflammation of reproductive or urinary tract
- Painful urination
- Itching, irritation
- Blisters
- Abdominal pain
- Warts in genital area

CAUSE

Bacterial, viral, or fungal infection

SCOPE

- Approximately 1,000,000 new cases of gonococcal disease are reported each year in the United States.
- 40–60% of children have been exposed to herpes simplex by 5 years of age.
- Incidence of pelvic inflammatory disease is highest among women ages 15–25.

Diagnosis

QUESTIONS THE DOCTOR MAY ASK

- Unprotected sex?
- Discharge?
- Rash?
- Joint pain?
- Discharge from vagina or urethra?
- Abdominal pain?

WHAT THE DOCTOR LOOKS FOR

- Signs and symptoms of STD
- The diagnosis of suspected child sexual abuse must be considered in any child with an STD.
- The source of infection should be determined in all cases, if possible.
- Infection with other sexually transmitted diseases, including syphilis, chlamydia, trichomonas, and possibly human immunodeficiency virus (HIV), should be considered.

TESTS AND PROCEDURES

- Blood tests
- Culture of infectious fluids
- In suspected sexual abuse, genital, rectal, and pharyngeal cultures should be collected.

 ## Treatment

GENERAL MEASURES

- Antibiotic therapy
- Treatment of partners or contacts should be initiated in all cases.
- Most STDs must be reported to health authorities.
- Suspected cases of sexual abuse must be reported to law enforcement authorities.

ACTIVITY

N/A

DIET

N/A

 ## Medications

COMMONLY PRESCRIBED DRUGS

- Antibiotics
- Antiviral drugs

 ## Follow-Up

WHAT TO EXPECT

- Outcome depends on diagnosis.
- In many cases, infections can be effectively eradicated before the development of complications.
- Viral infections (e.g., herpes simplex) may be life-long and recur over time.

SIGNS TO WATCH

Persistence, worsening, or recurrence of symptoms

PREVENTION

The use of condoms prevents or decreases the risk of transmission of most STDs.

 ## Common Questions and Answers

Q: Will STDs lead to infertility problems?
A: Some cases will cause obstruction of fallopian tubes, which may cause infertility or tubal pregnancy.

Short Bowel Syndrome

 ## Basics

DESCRIPTION

Short bowel syndrome results from loss of bowel tissue which leads to malnutrition and fluid and electrolyte loss.

SIGNS AND SYMPTOMS

- Diarrhea
- Vomiting
- Weight loss
- Failure to thrive
- Dehydration

CAUSES

- Inflammation of bowel
- Peritonitis
- Twisting of bowel
- Obstruction
- Trauma

 ## Diagnosis

QUESTIONS THE DOCTOR MAY ASK

- Abdominal distention?
- Abdominal pain?
- Bone pain?
- Stooling pattern?
- Weight loss or gain?
- Medication history?
- Surgical history?

WHAT THE DOCTOR LOOKS FOR

- Physical examination
- Height and weight
- Surgical scar

TESTS AND PROCEDURES

X-ray studies

Treatment

GENERAL MEASURES

- Diet management
- Drug therapy
- Surgery may be necessary.

ACTIVITY

N/A

DIET

- Oral diet is recommended for those patients who are able to avoid intravenous nutrition or tube feeds. A low-lactose diet may be well tolerated. Low-oxalate diets are helpful in preventing oxalate stones.
- Fluid and salt balance
- Parenteral (intravenous) nutrition (PN)

Medications

COMMONLY PRESCRIBED DRUGS

- Vitamin and mineral supplementation
- H₂ antagonists
- Antidiarrheal drugs
- Cholestyramine
- Octreotide
- Antibiotics: metronidazole, trimethoprim-sul-famethoxazole, vancomycin, and gentamicin
- Cisapride

Follow-Up

WHAT TO EXPECT

- Depends on site and extent of bowel surgery
- Prognosis is markedly improved with parenteral nutrition.

SIGNS TO WATCH

Vomiting, diarrhea, weight loss, severe fluid and salt imbalance, severe infection, intestinal obstruction

PREVENTION

N/A

Common Questions and Answers

Q: What are the favorable prognostic factors in short bowel syndrome?
A: The more of the bowel resected the worse the prognosis. Loss of ICV, worsens prognosis. Loss of jejunum and ileum worsens than loss of colon. Longer it takes to tolerate full enteral feeds, worse the prognosis. Development of severe TPN liver disease: poor prognosis. Neonates have greater chances of bowel adaptation than adults.

Q: Are elemental formulas better than intact formulas in the management of patients with short bowel syndrome?
A: Recent studies have shown similar rates of absorption, stomal output, electrolyte losses between elemental and intact formulas. The disadvantages of elemental formulas include high osmolality and cost.

Sickle Cell Anemia

Basics

DESCRIPTION

Sickle cell anemia is an inherited disorder that causes red blood cells to be deformed. The elongated, sickle-shaped cells can block small blood vessels, causing painful "crises" as tissues and organs are deprived of oxygen. Complications include pain, inadequate supply of oxygen to bone, acute chest syndrome, stroke, increased risk of infection, and other conditions.

SIGNS AND SYMPTOMS

- Painful swelling of hands and/or feet in infants (dactylitis)
- Lethargy
- Pain (can occur in any part of the body)
- Warmth, tenderness, decreased range of motion at site of pain
- Fever
- Pallor
- Yellowing of the eyes (jaundice)
- Bed-wetting (enuresis)—very common
- Persistent erection (priapism)
- Blood in urine

CAUSES

Genetic defect; person must inherit two copies of the gene, one from each parent

SCOPE

- Eight percent of African Americans carry a copy of the sickle cell anemia gene.
- First pain symptoms occur at approximately 1 year of age.

Diagnosis

QUESTIONS THE DOCTOR MAY ASK

- Family history?
- Bone pain?
- Abdominal pain?
- Chest pain?
- Jaundice?
- Dark or bloody urine?
- Severity and extent of pain?
- Fever?

WHAT THE DOCTOR LOOKS FOR

- Painful swelling of fingers (dactylitis): Incidence is greatest during the first year of life.
- Severe infection: Risk is greatest during the first 6 years of life, and especially during the first 2 years of life.
- Acute chest syndrome—chest pain, cough, fever, abnormal chest X-ray
- Stroke: Peak age is 5–10 years, but can occur any time.
- Gallstones: Risk is greatest after 10 years of age.
- High-risk pregnancy: All vascular complications of sickle cell disease are worsened by pregnancy.
- It is often difficult to distinguish sickle cell crisis from concurrent infectious disease, complications, and psychologic factors.

TESTS AND PROCEDURES

- Screening test: sickledex
- Blood tests
- Bone scan and bone marrow scan
- Chest x-ray
- Abdominal ultrasound
- Computed tomography (CT), magnetic resonance imaging (MRI), arteriogram if stroke suspected

Treatment

GENERAL MEASURES

- Prevention of infection with antibiotics, vaccine
- Folic acid supplementation
- Attention to good oral hydration
- Parental monitoring for:
  - Fever
  - Enlarged spleen
  - Pain
  - Increased jaundice
- Treatment of fever
- Treatment of pain

Sickle Cell Anemia

- Comfort measures (massage, heating pad, warm soaks)
- Oral (non-narcotic) analgesics, escalating to narcotic analgesics
- Management of other medical conditions (acute chest syndrome)
- Blood transfusions as needed

DIET

Normal for age

ACTIVITY

No absolute restrictions, but some activities may lead to pain episodes (e.g., heavy lifting, strenuous sports, swimming in cold water).

Medications

COMMONLY PRESCRIBED DRUGS

Drugs for pain relief and preventive antibiotics are usually prescribed.

Follow-Up

WHAT TO EXPECT

- Recurrences of fever, pain
- Blood in urine
- Development of gallstones
- Younger children (less than 1 year old) are seen more frequently.
- Regular blood tests, monthly transfusions may be needed

SIGNS TO WATCH

- Signs and symptoms of infection (especially fever)
- Spleen disorder (parents learn to palpate spleen)

- Increased destruction of red blood cells or pallor
- Stroke

PREVENTION

N/A

Common Questions and Answers

Q: Will the child live to be an adult?
A: The life expectancy of children with sickle cell disease has improved dramatically over the past decade. The average life expectancy for a person with sickle cell disease is over 50 years and is expected to improve as therapy for the disease improves.

Q: Will the child always be small and skinny?
A: There is quite a bit to learn about the nutritional requirements of children with sickle cell disease. It has been observed, however, that many of the children are slender. Adults with sickle cell disease are on average the same size as adults without sickle cell disease. Although children with sickle cell disease go through their growth spurt (and experience puberty) later than their peers, they will have a growth spurt and ultimately be of a normal height.

Q: Is there any cure for sickle cell disease?
A: Bone marrow transplantation (BMT) is the only known cure for sickle cell disease. BMT requires destroying all the bone marrow of the child with sickle cell disease with strong drugs and/or radiation and replacing it with the bone marrow of a person without sickle cell disease. It is done rarely because the side effects of the BMT are serious and include death. At this time, the procedure itself is thought to be worse than the disease.

Q: What triggers or starts off a pain episode?
A: Some children say that changes in the weather (e.g., hot to cold or vice versa) bring on pain episodes. Others say that jumping into a swimming pool or the ocean bring on pain. Trauma (e.g., being tackled on the football field) can also bring on pain. But in the majority of cases, there is no known cause.

Sinusitis

 ## Basics

DESCRIPTION

Sinusitis is inflammation of the nasal sinuses. It may be acute or chronic depending on duration of infection. Sinusitis occurs when pus accumulates in the sinus.

SIGNS AND SYMPTOMS

- Nasal congestion
- Gradual buildup of pressure sinus area with tenderness
- Nasal discharge
- Malaise
- Sore throat (sometimes)
- Headache
- Fever
- Pain over cheeks and upper teeth, worse with bending or leaning forward
- Pain over eyebrows
- Pain over eyes
- Pain behind eyes
- Cough (occasional)
- Postnasal drip
- Swelling around eyes
- Symptoms aggravated by air travel

CAUSES

Bacterial, viral, or fungal infection

SCOPE

Sinusitis is a complication of approximately 5–10% of upper respiratory tract infections.

 ## Diagnosis

QUESTIONS THE DOCTOR MAY ASK

- Does it hurt to lean forward?
- Fever?
- Pain in face?
- Recent infection?
- Headache?
- Post nasal drip?

WHAT THE DOCTOR LOOKS FOR

- Tenderness over sinuses
- Swollen nasal passage
- Source of fever
- Drainage in nose or throat

TESTS AND PROCEDURES

- Transillumination: using light to visualize sinuses
- Sample of sinus fluid
- Culture for microbiological analysis
- Sweat salt test
- Sinus biopsy
- X-ray of skull
- Computed tomography (CT)

 ## Treatment

GENERAL MEASURES

- Humidifier
- Surgery may be recommended.

ACTIVITY

N/A

DIET

N/A

Medications

COMMONLY PRESCRIBED DRUGS

- Amoxicillin
- Amoxicillin/clavulanate
- Erythromycin/sulfisoxazole
- Amoxicillin and sulfisoxazole
- Normal saline: squirt into each nostril once or twice daily
- Decongestants
- Guaifenesin
- Topical nasal steroids

 ## Follow-Up

WHAT TO EXPECT

- Improvement of acute sinusitis should be seen within 3 to 4 days after starting antibiotics.
- Up to 45% of cases of acute sinusitis children resolve spontaneously.
- Prognosis is excellent for those who are otherwise healthy.

SIGNS TO WATCH

Persistence of symptoms that do not respond to therapy

PREVENTION

- Preventive antibiotics
- Avoid allergen exposure and treat allergies if present.
- Practice daily nasal hygiene through the use of normal saline drops/spray.
- Increase ambient humidity with a humidifier.

 ## Common Questions and Answers

Q: Are all of the sinuses present at birth?
A: No, the maxillary and ethmoid sinuses form during the second trimester of gestation and are present at birth. They continue to enlarge until the preteen years. The frontal sinuses are present at age 5–6 years and are not completely developed until late adolescence.

Q: Does the nasal discharge seen with sinusitis have to be purulent and thick?
A: No. Though the nasal discharge is often described as purulent and thick, it may also be clear or mucoid. It may be thick or thin.

Q: Are radiographs useful in the diagnosis of sinusitis?
A: This is a controversial subject. Radiographs should be used in conjunction with clinical suspicion and should be used when signs and symptoms are not clear cut. In the absence of symptoms, it is difficult to make a radiographic diagnosis of sinusitis.

Slipped Capital Femoral Epipysis

 Basics

DESCRIPTION

Slipped capitus femoral is the dislocation of the end of the femur, the long bone of the thigh.

SIGNS AND SYMPTOMS

- Pain in hip or knee
- Limited range of motion
- Abnormal movement of extremity
- Limp or abnormal gait
- Atrophy of thigh muscle

CAUSE

Undetermined; may be due to multiple factors

SCOPE

- More common in males
- Age of onset in males is 14–16 years; in females, 11–13 years (essentially never after onset of menstruation).
- Associated with obesity, increased height, genital underdevelopment, pituitary tumors

 Diagnosis

QUESTIONS THE DOCTOR MAY ASK

- Pain in hip or knee?
- History of trauma?
- Growth pattern/growth spurt?
- Difficulty walking?

WHAT THE DOCTOR LOOKS FOR

- Occasional history of trauma
- Tenderness in hip
- Pain in knee
- Gait
- Joint movement

TESTS AND PROCEDURES

- X-rays
- Blood tests

Treatment

GENERAL MEASURES

- Therapy intended to prevent complications and further slipping
- Conservative: bed rest with traction
- Manipulative reduction
- Surgery may be recommended.

ACTIVITY

Requires bed rest initially

DIET

N/A

 ## Medications

COMMONLY PRESCRIBED DRUGS

N/A

 ## Follow-Up

WHAT TO EXPECT

- Most recover after treatment
- Can have damage to bone to slow linear growth

SIGNS TO WATCH

Recurrence of pain

PREVENTION

N/A

 ## Common Questions and Answers

Q: Is this problem a result of obesity?
A: This was formerly the explanation, but there are many conditions associated with slipped capital femoral epipysis.

Sore Throat

 Basics

DESCRIPTION

Sore throat, or pharyngitis, is an inflammation of the pharynx (throat) most commonly caused by acute infection by a virus, bacteria, or fungi.

SIGNS AND SYMPTOMS

- Sore throat
- Enlarged tonsils
- Enlarged lymph nodes in neck
- Absence of cough; hoarseness, lower respiratory symptoms
- Fever over 102.5°F (39.1°C)
- Rash
- Loss of appetite
- Chills
- Malaise
- Headache
- Reddened eyes

CAUSES

- Bacterial (streptococcus, staphylococcus), viral, or fungal infection
- Chronic: noninfectious; chemical irritation; smoking; cancer

SCOPE

- An estimated 30 million cases of sore throat are diagnosed yearly in the United States.
- Viral disease is more common in younger children, especially in cold winter months.
- Day-care attendance increases frequency of disease.

 Diagnosis

QUESTIONS THE DOCTOR MAY ASK

- Been swimming in an inadequately chlorinated pool?
- Travel to the former Soviet Union?
- Ingestion of undercooked meat or handling rabbits?

WHAT THE DOCTOR LOOKS FOR

- Characteristic signs and symptoms of sore throat
- Enlarged lymph nodes
- Other conditions associated with sore throat

TESTS AND PROCEDURES

- Throat swab for microbiological analysis
- Blood tests

 Treatment

GENERAL MEASURES

- Usually no therapy indicated except for bacterial infection
- Gargling with warm-hot salt water; effective symptomatic relief

ACTIVITY

N/A

DIET

N/A

MEDICATIONS

COMMONLY PRESCRIBED DRUGS

- Antibiotics for bacterial infection: penicillin, erythromycin, amoxicillin, clindamycin
- Acetaminophen

 Follow-Up

WHAT TO EXPECT

- Almost always acute and self-limited, lasting 4–14 days, depending on cause
- Prognosis is excellent.
- Few suffer complications from bacterial disease.
- Rare deaths from rupture of the spleen

SIGNS TO WATCH

Worsening of symptoms

PREVENTION

- Prompt treatment leads to fewer secondary cases of streptococcal disease.
- Preventive penicillin is recommended by some for children with recurring bacterial disease with history of acute rheumatic fever.
- Immunization with diphtheria toxoid

 Common Questions and Answers

Q: How soon can children with streptococcal pharyngitis return to school or day care?
A: When they are without fever, and after at least 24 hours of therapy.

Spinal Muscular Atrophy

 Basics

DESCRIPTION

Spinal muscular atrophy (SMA) is a nerve disorder that causes progressive weakness; death due to respiratory failure is common. It is one of the causes of "floppy infant syndrome."

SIGNS AND SYMPTOMS

- Weak muscle tone
- Generalized weakness
- Poor head control
- Missed or delayed developmental milestones
- Breathing difficulties from neurologic defects
- Respiratory failure

CAUSES

Unknown; hereditary disorder

SCOPE

Worldwide incidence is approximately 1 per 4000 live births (although areas with higher incidence have been identified), making SMA one of the most common lethal hereditary disorders in humans.

 Diagnosis

QUESTIONS THE DOCTOR MAY ASK

- Development?
- Head control?
- Family history of "floppy infants"?
- Breathing problems?

WHAT THE DOCTOR LOOKS FOR

- Twitching of tongue
- Weakness of muscles
- Absent deep tendon reflexes
- Poor head control
- Shallow breathing

TESTS AND PROCEDURES

- Electromyography
- Muscle biopsy
- Blood tests

Treatment

GENERAL MEASURES

- No effective therapy for spinal muscle atrophy
- Supportive/anticipatory care directed toward respiratory complications, postural support, and genetic counseling

ACTIVITY

N/A

DIET

N/A

 ## Medications

COMMONLY PRESCRIBED DRUGS

N/A

 ## Follow-Up

WHAT TO EXPECT

- Anticipatory/preventive medical issues: respiratory condition, physical therapy to prevent contractures, etc.
- Ongoing planning and counseling regarding prognosis and appropriate medical intervention
- Follow-up genetic counseling

SIGNS TO WATCH

A seemingly minor respiratory infection calls for close monitoring and follow-up because it may rapidly become serious.

PREVENTION

N/A

 ## Common Questions and Answers

Q: Can routine vaccinations be given to infants with SMA?
A: Yes. In addition to routine vaccinations, yearly influenza vaccinations are recommended for older children with quadriplegia because they are at high risk for common respiratory illnesses.

Stool Soiling

 Basics

DESCRIPTION

Stool soiling, or encopresis, is overflow incontinence resulting from chronic constipation.

SIGNS AND SYMPTOMS

- Constipation, usually
- Pasty stool found on underclothes
- Fecal or foul odor surrounding the child
- Pain around the navel
- Occasional passage of a large volume of stool
- History of painful bowel movements
- Shyness and withdrawal, acting out, or aggressive behavior
- Some children with stool soiling have had psychotherapy.
- Some have had recurrent urinary tract infections.

CAUSES

- Psychologic (toilet training issues)
- Rectal disorders (e.g., painful defecation, poor muscle tone)
- Dietary or metabolic (lack of fiber, excessive protein or milk intake, inadequate water intake, hypothyroidism)

SCOPE

- Encopresis affects 1.3% of all children over 4 years of age.
- It is approximately 6 times more common in boys than girls.
- No association with family size, position in the family, age of parents, or socioeconomic status

 Diagnosis

QUESTIONS THE DOCTOR MAY ASK

- Diet
- Toilet training procedure
- Disclipine techniques
- Typical stooling pattern
- Social problems
- Urinary tract infections, especially in girls
- Abdominal discomfort
- Decreased appetite

WHAT THE DOCTOR LOOKS FOR

- The physician must determine if stool leakage is caused by functional constipation or an underlying anatomic, metabolic, or endocrinologic abnormality.

TESTS AND PROCEDURES

Usually none—at times, barium enema

 Treatment

GENERAL MEASURES

- Management combines pharmacology, behavioral modification, and dietary alterations.
- Remove fecal impaction.
- Stool softener
- Decrease family stress.
- Have child sit on toilet for 5 to 10 minutes one to two times per day (tailored to the age of the child).
- Delay toilet training if the child is in diapers (to reduce stress).
- Motivate.
- Biofeedback (reserved for very difficult cases)

ACTIVITY

N/A

DIET

- High-fiber diet
- Adequate fluid

Medications

COMMONLY PRESCRIBED DRUGS

Enemas, cathartic regimens including laxatives

 Follow-Up

WHAT TO EXPECT

- The first follow-up is at 2 weeks to ensure compliance and success with the initial management.
- If the fecal impaction has been removed successfully, then a reward system is started.
- The patient is observed at monthly intervals to ensure motivation and to be supportive.
- Treatment with stool softeners is needed until behavior and diet have improved.
- Medication is often needed for 6 months or longer.

SIGNS TO WATCH

- Lack of improvement
- Change in personality
- Good growth pattern

PREVENTION

- Parents may think that their child's soiling is deliberate. The child can neither feel the passage of stool nor prevent it.
- Patients or their parents often stop stool softeners as soon as a normal stool pattern starts. If therapy has been ended prematurely, the patient's constipation and encopresis returns immediately.

 Common Questions and Answers

Q: Is the medicine addictive?
A: Stool softeners rather than cathartics are chosen for long-term therapy because the colon does not become dependent.

Q: Will my child become sick if this problem is not resolved?
A: Most children with chronic constipation and encopresis grow well and do not develop other health problems. The major problems are social and should be taken seriously. Social development is crucial for the school-aged child.

Stuttering

 ## Basics

DESCRIPTION

Stuttering is the repetition of short speech segments (fractions of a word) or the inability to initiate a word (blockage). It is associated with signs of physical distress, such as a facial grimace, tonic jaw tension, or change in respiratory rate.

- It should not be confused with transient loss in normal rate and rhythm of speech between the ages of 2.5 to 4 years; repetition is usually of whole words (e.g., I want . . . I want) and is not associated with any signs of subjective stress in the child.

SIGNS AND SYMPTOMS

- Repetition of short speech segments
- Inability to initiate words
- Facial grimace
- Jaw tension
- Change in respiratory rate

CAUSES

- Unknown; probably multiple factors
- May stem from lack of development of area in brain relative to speech
- May be psychological problem
- Stress

SCOPE

- Stuttering affects 1–2% of the general population.
- Four times more common in males
- Strong familial tendency

 ## Diagnosis

QUESTIONS THE DOCTOR MAY ASK

- Speech development?
- Family's attempt to correct speech?
- Social adjustment?
- Academic record?
- Age of onset?
- Frequency, severity, and type of stuttering?
- Signs of physical tension?
- Parental reaction?
- Family history?
- Developmental history?

WHAT THE DOCTOR LOOKS FOR

- Physical examination
- Development assessment
- Speech pattern
- Neurologic examination

TESTS AND PROCEDURES

Speech therapy evaluation

 ## Treatment

GENERAL MEASURES

Early referral to speech therapist is essential.

ACTIVITY

N/A

DIET

N/A

Medications

COMMONLY PRESCRIBED DRUGS

N/A

 Follow-Up

WHAT TO EXPECT

- Improvement is gradual in first year of speech therapy, depending on the age at intervention.
- 75% of preschool stutterers have partial or complete remission during elementary school.
- Prognosis for remission is less hopeful if a parent or sibling stutters.
- Adolescent stutterer often improves gradually with physical and emotional maturity; final state usually includes fluent speech, except for stuttering with excitement or stress, throughout adulthood.
- Best performance occurs with whispering, speaking foreign languages, reading aloud in privacy, and building confidence over time.

SIGNS TO WATCH

Severe social maladjustment, poor school performance

PREVENTION

N/A

 Common Questions and Answers

Q: Do preschoolers who have what appears to be only physiologic dysfluency require therapy?
A: No. Physiologic dysfluency resolves with time.

Q: Do people who stutter have a higher frequency of learning disabilities?
A: No. Stutterers do, in fact, have worse school performance overall, but this is believed to be caused by low self-esteem and social maladjustment. A major goal of early therapy is to minimize the impact of the stuttering on other aspects of the child's life.

Q: Is stuttering associated with Tourrette syndrome?
A: Although the two problems share some common features, the disorders have not been shown to be linked.

Stye

Basics

DESCRIPTION

Stye, or hordeolum, is an inflammation or infection of the eyelid margin, often involving the hair follicles of the eyelashes.

SIGNS AND SYMPTOMS

- Redness of the edge of the eyelid with peeling, weeping
- Inflammation of the eyelashes
- Itching or peeling of the eyelids, chronic redness, eye irritation leading to tenderness and pain

CAUSES

- The most common cause of eyelid infection is staphylococcal infection, although other organisms may also be involved.
- Seborrhea can predispose to infections of the eyelid.

SCOPE

Extremely common

Diagnosis

QUESTIONS THE DOCTOR MAY ASK

- Symptoms worse on awakening?
- Difficulty opening eye?
- Other staph infection in skin?
- Treatment?
- Presence of skin rashes?

WHAT THE DOCTOR LOOKS FOR

- Partial loss of eyelashes
- Dried exudate on eye loss
- Visual activity
- Small abscesses

TESTS AND PROCEDURES

N/A

Treatment

GENERAL MEASURES

- Warm compresses on the area of inflammation can help increase blood supply and promote healing.
- Cleanse the eyelids using a solution of tap water and baby shampoo or a commercially prepared hypoallergenic cleanser.
- The stye should not be squeezed.
- Good personal hygiene with attention to cleansing the eyelids on a daily basis to prevent recurrent infections
- Application of an antibiotic ointment (such as erythromycin) to the margin of the eyelid after proper cleansing (except children under 12, where there is a risk of vision problems). This helps reduce bacterial growth.
- Minor surgery may be required to drain infection.

ACTIVITY

No restrictions

DIET

No special diet

Medications

COMMONLY PRESCRIBED DRUGS

- Erythromycin ophthalmic ointment
- Aminoglycoside ophthalmic ointment (gentamicin)

 ## Follow-Up

WHAT TO EXPECT

Responds well to treatment, but tends to recur in some patients

SIGNS TO WATCH

N/A

PREVENTION

Eyelid hygiene

 ## Common Questions and Answers

Q: Which patients are prone to recurrent styes?
A: Those with allergies and seborrhea.

Sudden Infant Death Syndrome (SIDS)

 Basics

DESCRIPTION

Sudden infant death syndrome (SIDS) is the sudden and unexpected death of an infant under 1 year of age which remains unexplained after a thorough case investigation, including performance of a complete autopsy, examination of the death scene, and review of the clinical history. Apparent life threatening events (ALTEs) are a related entity and increase the risk of SIDS.

SIGNS AND SYMPTOMS

These babies generally appear healthy, or may have had a minor upper respiratory or gastrointestinal infection in the last 2 weeks of life.

CAUSES

- There are many theories about the cause of SIDS. There may be subtle developmental abnormalities resulting from brain injury.
- Possible causes:
  ▸ Abnormal respiratory control
  ▸ Upper airway obstruction
  ▸ Nervous system abnormalities
  ▸ Irregular heart rhythms
  ▸ Carbon dioxide rebreathing in face-down position on soft surface
- SIDS may occur when a combination of factors coincide; such triggers may include infectious agents, climatic changes, or environmental factors.

SCOPE

- There are approximately 4700 cases of SIDS annually in the United States.
- 1.4 cases per 1000 live births
- 90% of cases occur before 6 months of age

 Diagnosis

QUESTIONS THE DOCTOR MAY ASK

- When was the last time the baby was seen alive?
- Where was the baby found?
- In what position was the baby found?
- What was the child wearing?
- Were there blankets, stuffed toys, or bumpers at the baby's head?
- Any recent illnesses?
- Prenatal history?
- History of previous maternal miscarriages?
- Date of last immunizations?
- Prior medical problems?
- Prior history of apnea?

WHAT THE DOCTOR LOOKS FOR

- Evidence of trauma
- Congenital malformation

TESTS AND PROCEDURES

- Autopsy
- X-rays
- Blood tests

 Treatment

GENERAL MEASURES

- The medical examiner or coroner's office should be notified of all SIDS deaths.
- Referral to a SIDS center
- SIDS deaths have a powerful impact on families and their functioning. Health care providers can play an important role in providing immediate information about SIDS and sensitive counseling to limit parents' misinformation and feelings of guilt.

Sudden Infant Death Syndrome (SIDS)

- Counseling needs of families vary from short-term to long-term; support groups are helpful to many couples. Providers should be familiar with resources available in their communities to help families mourning a SIDS death. Parents need to be counseled about subsequent pregnancies.
- Follow-up counseling, including review of the autopsy report with the family after some time has passed, is important to help understand this condition and to clear the tremendous guilt these families experience.

ACTIVITY

N/A

DIET

N/A

 Follow-Up

WHAT TO EXPECT

N/A

SIGNS TO WATCH

N/A

PREVENTION

- Because a SIDS death is sudden and the cause is unknown, SIDS cannot be "treated." However, there are some measures that may be effective in preventing SIDS:
  - Maternal avoidance of cigarette and illicit drug use during pregnancy
  - Breast-feeding
  - Avoid letting the baby sleep on his or her stomach.
  - Avoid excessive bed clothing and soft bedding.
  - Avoid passive cigarette smoke exposure.
- Recent studies suggest significant risk reduction when baby is placed on the back or side for sleep. Because infants placed on their side may turn over during sleep onto their stomach, it is now believed that back position is best.
- Apnea monitors for infants with apparent life-threatening episodes

 Common Questions and Answers

Q: Do all infants who die suddenly and unexpectedly require an autopsy?
A: Yes, it is estimated that autopsy reveals a cause of death in approximately 15% of "SIDS" deaths. The diagnosis of SIDS cannot be made without an autopsy.

Q: Does SIDS run in families?
A: Large, controlled studies indicate no increased risk of SIDS in subsequent siblings.

Suicide

 ## Basics

DESCRIPTION

Suicide is the act of intentionally trying to kill oneself or succeeding in killing oneself. Suicidal thoughts or gestures should be taken seriously and treated appropriately.

SIGNS AND SYMPTOMS

N/A

CAUSES

- Final act of depression and/or resignation
- Impulsive act designed to punish caregivers/significant others
- Help-seeking gesture

SCOPE

- Suicide rate for persons ages 15–19 in 1992: 10.9 per 100,000
- Rate for ages 10–14 in 1992: 1.7 per 100,000
- Third leading cause of death among males 15–24
- Fourth leading cause of death among females 15–24
- Rate currently greatest for white males
- Rates increasing fastest for black males
- Estimated ratio of suicide attempts: completions range from 50 to 200:1.
- Male-to-female ratio for completed suicides 3:1.
- Male-to-female ratio for attempted suicides 1:3 (males use more lethal means and may have fewer "gestures").
- Preadolescents rarely attempt suicide; they perceive death as reversible.
- Ingestions used in 15 to 20% of male and 25 to 30% of female completed suicides; common in suicide attempts and gestures; many go unreported.
- Guns and hanging are most lethal methods; firearms used in 60% of male and 40% of female completed suicides, whereas hangings and strangulation are used in 15 to 20% of male and 10% of female completed suicides.

 ## Diagnosis

QUESTIONS THE DOCTOR MAY ASK

- Circumstances of suicide attempt?
- Estimation of amount of drug ingested?
- Seriousness of attempt (e.g., method, lethality, other circumstances)?
- Risk for repeat attempt?
- Predisposing factors (e.g., substance abuse, chronic disease, mental illness)?
- Psychological status (e.g., depression, hopelessness, impulsiveness, low self-esteem)?

WHAT THE DOCTOR LOOKS FOR

- Physical examination
  - Blood pressure, pulse
  - Evidence of drug effects
  - Eye examination—pupil size
  - Breathing problems
  - Abdominal pain
  - Evidence of pregnancy

TESTS AND PROCEDURES

- Drug tests
- Pregnancy test (if female)
- Blood tests
- Abdominal x-ray

 ## Treatment

GENERAL MEASURES

- Provide first aid as needed, including rescue breathing.
- Bring remaining pills, available drugs/pharmaceuticals, etc., along to hospital.
- Intensive monitoring
- Hospitalization may be required.

ACTIVITY

N/A

DIET

N/A

Medications

COMMONLY PRESCRIBED DRUGS

- Charcoal, naloxone, and flumazenil
- Antidepressants
- Phenothiazines

 Follow-Up

WHAT TO EXPECT

- Patients often need long-term care and often show slow improvement.
- 20–50% of adolescents who attempt suicide make a repeat attempt.
- Best predictors of repeat attempt: male gender, method other than ingestion

SIGNS TO WATCH

- Acute life stressors (pregnancy, fights with peers, parents)
- Failure to comply with mental health follow-up
- Withdrawal
- Sudden sense of resolution; patients may become calmer when they have determined to end their life

PREVENTION

Eliminate easy access to firearms.

 Common Questions and Answers

Q: If I ask the questions about suicide directly, might I offend the person or put the idea in his/her head?
A: No. They are usually relieved to have a caring person with whom to talk. There is danger in raising the question only if you do nothing with the answer. Appropriate referral to supportive mental health services saves lives.

Swimmer's Ear

 Basics

DESCRIPTION

Swimmer's ear, or otitis externa, is an inflammation of the external ear canal. It may be caused by infection with bacteria or a fungus. It is often associated with swimming because moisture becomes trapped in the outer ear canal and provides an appropriate environment (i.e., warm and moist) for the growth of bacteria and fungi.

SIGNS AND SYMPTOMS

- Itching
- Plugging of the ear
- Pain
- Reddening
- Discharge of pus
- Eczema of ear

CAUSES

- Trauma
- Infection (bacterial, fungal)
- Skin disorders (e.g., eczema, seborrhea)

SCOPE

Highest incidence during summer months

 Diagnosis

QUESTIONS THE DOCTOR MAY ASK

- Ear pain?
- Discharge from ear?

WHAT THE DOCTOR LOOKS FOR

- Risk factors of swimmer's ear
- Characteristic signs and symptoms of swimmer's ear
- Pain when the ear is pulled

TESTS AND PROCEDURES

Culture and microbiologic analysis

Treatment

GENERAL MEASURES

Pain relievers, if needed

ACTIVITY

N/A

DIET

N/A

 ## Medications

COMMONLY PRESCRIBED DRUGS

- Analgesics
- Antibiotics

 ## Follow-Up

WHAT TO EXPECT

- Improvement within 24 to 48 hours of beginning antibiotics
- Prognosis is excellent.

SIGNS TO WATCH

- Fever
- Severe inflammation, especially in a person with an impaired immune system

PREVENTION

Acetic acid drops in ears after swimming or immersion of the ears help prevent microbial growth in the ear.

 ## Common Questions and Answers

Q: How long should one avoid swimming?
A: Until resolution of infection; then use acetic acid ear drops for prevention.

Tear Duct Obstruction

Basics

DESCRIPTION

A tear duct obstruction is a blockage of the portion of the tear drainage system extending from the eye to the nose. It may lead to infection of the tear system.

SIGNS AND SYMPTOMS

- Excessive tearing
- Crusting of eyelashes, particularly upon awaking
- Red eye
- Discharge from eye

CAUSES

Congenital obstruction of duct from eye to nose

SCOPE

Tear duct obstruction affects approximately 5% of newborns.

Diagnosis

QUESTIONS THE DOCTOR MAY ASK

- Excessive tearing?
- Reddened area under lower eyelid?
- Eye discharge?

WHAT THE DOCTOR LOOKS FOR

Signs and symptoms of tear duct obstruction

TESTS

Dye disappearance test

Treatment

GENERAL MEASURES

- Initially, tear sac massage and either oph-thalmic antibiotic drops or ointment are applied when eye discharge increases.
- If symptomatic at 12 months of age, probing and irrigation may be performed.
- Surgery may be performed.

ACTIVITY

N/A

DIET

N/A

 ## Medications

COMMONLY PRESCRIBED DRUGS

Ophthalmic antibiotic

 ## Follow-Up

WHAT TO EXPECT

- Spontaneous resolution in approximately 95% of patients by 12 months of age
- Patients should be reevaluated at 12 months of age.

SIGNS TO WATCH

N/A

PREVENTION

N/A

 ## Common Questions and Answers

Q: Is my child in any danger while the duct remains obstructed?
A: Occasionally, the contents of the sac can become infected and require antibiotics.

Q: Why not wait longer to do the probing and irrigation?
A: The failure rate of the initial procedure increases with age: if performed before 13 months of age 96% success rate, between 13 and 18 months of age 77% success rate, and between 18 and 24 months 54% success rate.

Tendinitis

 ## Basics

DESCRIPTION

Tendinitis is the inflammation of a tendon, which may affect adjacent areas.

SIGNS AND SYMPTOMS

- Pain over the point of inflammation, usually worsened by active motion but may be present at rest
- Tenderness over the affected tendon
- Mild reddening and increased heat of overlying skin

CAUSES

Usually related to repetitive activity or trauma, but can occur without obvious cause

SCOPE

- Incidence increases with age and at time of puberty.
- There may be a slight increase in incidence in girls.

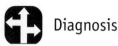 ## Diagnosis

QUESTIONS THE DOCTOR MAY ASK

- Athletics or chronic use?
- Computer use?
- Was a pop or snap felt at the time of the event?
- History of trauma or overuse?

WHAT THE DOCTOR LOOKS FOR

- Signs and symptoms of tendinitis
- Tenderness over tendon or bony prominence
- Evidence of trauma
- Bruises

TESTS AND PROCEDURES

- Blood tests
- X-rays

Treatment

GENERAL MEASURES

Relieve pain, reduce inflammation, rest the joint

ACTIVITY

- In acute phases, the involved muscle and tendon should be rested. Use slings and splints for the upper extremity. Use braces, canes, and/or crutches for the lower limbs.
- Physical therapy, once patient is free of pain

DIET

N/A

 ## Medications

COMMONLY PRESCRIBED DRUGS

Nonsteroidal anti-inflammatory drugs (NSAIDS)

 ## Follow-Up

WHAT TO EXPECT

- Improvement often takes 2–6 weeks.
- Prognosis is usually good for children; however, many of them suffer recurrences if proper exercises before desired activity are not performed.

SIGNS TO WATCH

If the provocative activity is resumed too soon, the irritation recurs.

PREVENTION

N/A

 ## Common Questions and Answers

Q: Which activities can result in overuse syndromes and tendinitis?
A: Virtually any repetitive activity in which children engage can cause tendinitis. For example, pain in the tendons of the thumb has occurred in children overusing video games.

Tetanus

Basics

DESCRIPTION

Tetanus is a disease characterized by spasms of the skeletal muscles and occasionally the throat due to toxin produced by the bacteria *Clostridium tetani*.

SIGNS AND SYMPTOMS

- Irregular, rapid, or slow heart rate
- Asphyxiation
- Convulsions
- Bluish discoloration around lips, eyes, and nail beds (cyanosis)
- Drooling, difficulty swallowing
- Fever
- Excessive thirst
- Irritability
- Muscular rigidity, spasms
- Stiff neck
- Pain at wound site

CAUSE

Toxin produced by *C. tetani*, an organism found in soil and as part of the normal intestinal flora in many domesticated animals, rats, and humans. Incubation is 3–21 days.

SCOPE

- In the United States, there are 50–200 cases reported annually, including occasional cases of neonatal tetanus.
- About two-thirds of cases in the United States occur between May and November. People from rural areas and who are involved in agriculture are more likely to have contact with the organisms, although many cases are reported among intravenous drug abusers.

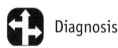

Diagnosis

QUESTIONS THE DOCTOR MAY ASK

- Injury that cuts skin?
- Painful muscles?
- Immunization history?
- Difficulty in swallowing?
- Breathing problems?

WHAT THE DOCTOR LOOKS FOR

- Tetanus-prone wound
- Muscle contractions
- Drooling
- Urinary retention
- Difficulty in moving facial muscles
- "Sardonic Smile"
- Spasms of muscles—"tetanic seizures"

TESTS AND PROCEDURES

- Blood tests
- Culture of wound for microbiological analysis

Treatment

GENERAL MEASURES

- All wounds should be cleaned thoroughly with soap and water, and foreign bodies should be sought aggressively and removed.
- Surgical removal of dead tissue and foreign bodies from the infected wound must be undertaken.
- If a wound is gangrenous, amputation may be necessary.
- Patients suspected of having tetanus should be rapidly transferred to an appropriate care center.
- Patients should be kept in a quiet, darkened room with minimum stimulus. Cardiac and respiratory status should be monitored closely.
- Tracheostomy may be necessary.

ACTIVITY

N/A

DIET

Parenteral (intravenous) nutrition is usually required to maintain adequate nutrition and hydration.

Medications

COMMONLY PRESCRIBED DRUGS

- Diazepam, chlorpromazine
- Vecuronium
- Human tetanus immune globulin (TIG)
- Tetanus antitoxin (TAT)
- Penicillin, tetracycline, vancomycin
- Beta-blockers

 ## Follow-Up

WHAT TO EXPECT

- With advances in the ability to provide respiratory support in an intensive care setting, the prognosis has improved markedly.
- Overall mortality rates have decreased from approximately 66% in the 1950s in the United States to 30% in the 1980s.
- Children and young adults have a much better prognosis than older individuals.
- In the absence of complications, recovery is usually complete in survivors without long-term effects.
- Signs and symptoms usually progress for approximately 1 week after presentation before reaching their worst. The patient's condition then plateaus for about 1 week and then gradually improves over 2 to 6 weeks.

SIGNS TO WATCH

N/A

PREVENTION

Immunization with tetanus toxoid. Diphtheria-pertussis-tetanus (DPT) vaccine is given at age 2 months, 4 months, 6 months, 15–18 months, and 4–6 years. A tetanus "booster" shot should be given at 14 to 16 years of age and every 10 years thereafter.

 ## Common Questions and Answers

Q: What is a tetanus-prone wound?
A: Deep puncture wounds and wounds causing a large amount of tissue death, including crushing wounds, large ragged lacerations, and wounds clearly contaminated with soil or feces. All wounds, including minor wounds such as corneal abrasions, insect bites, small lacerations, and burns, may be infected and lead to the development of tetanus.

Q: If the last tetanus shot was given 2 years ago, is another tetanus shot needed if there was a recent cut?
A: If all three tetanus shots were given, there is no need to give another. If the wound is minor, another is needed if last tetanus was 10 years ago. If wound is dirty or tetanus-prone and last shot was more than 5 years ago, another shot should be given.

Thalassemia

 ## Basics

DESCRIPTION

Thalassemia is a form of anemia caused by an inherited defect of hemoglobin, a protein that carries oxygen in red blood cells.

SIGNS AND SYMPTOMS

- Pallor
- Failure to thrive
- Growth retardation
- Abdominal distention
- "Chipmunk face"
- Heart failure

CAUSES

Genetic defect. Patients with trait have no symptoms.

SCOPE

More common in Chinese, Malaysian, Indochina, African, African-American, Mediterranean, Mid-Eastern, and Asian populations

 ## Diagnosis

QUESTIONS THE DOCTOR MAY ASK

- Family history of anemia?
- Paleness?
- Energy level?
- Growth record?
- Respiratory problems?

WHAT THE DOCTOR LOOKS FOR

- Paleness
- Cardiac enlargement
- Large liver or spleen

TESTS AND PROCEDURES

Blood tests

Treatment

GENERAL MEASURES

- Genetic counseling
- Folic acid supplementation
- Transfusion may be required.
- Chelation therapy
- Spleen may be surgically removed.
- Bone marrow transplantation may be recommended.

ACTIVITY

N/A

DIET

N/A

 ## Medications

COMMONLY PRESCRIBED DRUGS

Folic acid

 ## Follow-Up

WHAT TO EXPECT

N/A

SIGNS TO WATCH

- Decreased energy level
- Breathing problems
- Reduced exercise tolerance

PREVENTION

N/A

 ## Common Questions and Answers

Q: Is prenatal testing available?
A: Yes.

Q: What would be the optimal age for bone marrow transplant?
A: Optimal age would be around 5 years when they do not have evidence of iron overload.

Q: In a transfused patient when does iron overload become a problem and when is chelation started?
A: Usually after age of 5 years.

Toddler's Diarrhea

 Basics

DESCRIPTION

Toddler's diarrhea is chronic diarrhea lasting more than 3 weeks in a toddler with normal growth.

SIGNS AND SYMPTOMS

- Intermittant, watery, loose, or mushy stools may contain undigested food.
- Up to 6–10 stools a day
- No stooling at night
- Normal growth

CAUSES

- Motility disorder, i.e., irritable bowel syndrome of infancy
- Excessive fluid intake
- Diet low in fiber and fat

SCOPE

Toddler's diarrhea is the most common cause of diarrhea during the latter part of first year and the second year of life.

 Diagnosis

QUESTIONS THE DOCTOR MAY ASK

- Amount and type of fluids ingested during a 24-hour period?
- 24-hour diet recall?
- History of recent viral illness?
- Stool consistency, especially the first one passed in the morning?
- Recent weight loss?

WHAT THE DOCTOR LOOKS FOR

- Intermittent watery, loose, or mushy stools
- Toddlers can have 2–3 mushy stools to 6–10 watery stools per day.
- Stools are usually forceful and foul smelling.
- Can get diarrhea alternating with constipation or normal stools alternating with watery stools
- No stools are passed at night.
- First stool in the morning may have better consistency than those for the rest of the day.
- Normal growth unless put on a low-caloric diet to control the diarrhea
- Can see food particles because of rapid transit
- Physical examination—normal

TESTS AND PROCEDURES

- Blood tests
- Urinalysis
- Stool analysis

Treatment

GENERAL MEASURES

Dietary modification

ACTIVITY

N/A

DIET

- High-fat and low-carbohydrate diet
- Fluids need to be restricted.
- Fluids should consist of mainly milk.
- Juice intake needs to be decreased.
- High-fiber diet may be helpful.

 ## Medications

COMMONLY PRESCRIBED DRUGS

None required; may try a fiber supplement

 ## Follow-Up

WHAT TO EXPECT

- Improvement begins within days of changing fluid and food intake.
- Prognosis is good.

SIGNS TO WATCH

- Persistent diarrhea despite adherence to the prescribed diet
- Weight loss despite adequate intake
- Blood and mucus in diarrhea
- Loss of appetite, irritability, and vomiting

PREVENTION

N/A

 ## Common Questions and Answers

Q: Is growth normal in a patient with toddler's diarrhea?
A: Growth is normal.

Q: What are the components of a successful treatment plan?
A: Decreased fluid intake, increased fat intake, and possibly increased fiber intake

Toxoplasmosis

 ## Basics

DESCRIPTION

Toxoplasmosis is infection with the protozoan *Toxoplasma gondii*. There are four types of toxoplasmosis:
- Congenital toxoplasmosis: acute infection of mother during gestation that is passed to fetus
- Ocular toxoplasmosis: eye infection, usually resulting from congenital exposure but remaining latent until the second or third decade of life
- Acute toxoplasmosis in person with normal immune system
- Acute toxoplasmosis in person with immune deficiency: a life-threatening infection involving many organ systems such as heart, lung, liver, but especially the central nervous system

SIGNS AND SYMPTOMS

- 80–90% have no symptoms.
- Fever, malaise, night sweats, muscle ache
- Sore throat
- Rash
- Brain inflammation
- Paralysis of half the body, seizures, mental status changes
- Visual changes
- Heart, lung inflammation

CAUSES

- Exposure to *T. gondii*
- Congenital disease is passed from newly infected mother to fetus during pregnancy.
- Other syndromes may result from newly acquired infection or reactivation of latent infection.
- Ingestion of meats or foods containing eggs present in cat feces
- Infection can be transmitted by blood transfusion or organ transplantation.

SCOPE

- Affects more than 3500 newborns in the United States each year
- 70–90% of children with congenital toxoplasmosis have no symptoms at birth. Late effects occur in greater than 50% of untreated infants.

Diagnosis

QUESTIONS THE DOCTOR MAY ASK

- For acquired infection, history of contact with cats, eating raw or undercooked meat
- For congenital infection, history of maternal exposure

WHAT THE DOCTOR LOOKS FOR

- Physical examination
  - Swollen glands
  - Rash
  - Fever
  - Small bruises in skin
  - Eye examination
  - Calcification in X-ray of brain

TESTS AND PROCEDURES

- Screening of pregnant women and their infants in high-incidence areas
- Blood tests
- Computed tomography (CT) or magnetic resonance imaging (MRI)
- Hearing and vision tests
- Elevated liver function tests

 ## Treatment

GENERAL MEASURES

Medication

ACTIVITY

N/A

DIET

N/A

 ## Medications

COMMONLY PRESCRIBED DRUGS

- Pyrimethamine
- Sulfadiazine
- Folic acid

 ## Follow-Up

WHAT TO EXPECT

- The majority of acquired infections are asymptomatic or associated with mild short-lived symptoms.
- Majority of congenital infections have no symptoms, although late effects occur in greater than 50% of untreated infants.
- Symptomatic newborns are at significant risk for lasting effects, most frequently neurologic or ophthalmic.
- Prenatal treatment appears to decrease risk to newborn; therapy of all infected infants appears to improve outcome.

SIGNS TO WATCH

- Neurologic development
- Vision and hearing loss

PREVENTION

- Avoidance of undercooked meats
- Pregnant women need to exercise caution in caring for cats. Pregnant women should not clean litter boxes; if they must, wear rubber gloves and a disposable mask.

 ## Common Questions and Answers

Q: What is the risk of congenital infection in a mother with stable toxoplasmosis?
A: The risk of congenital infection in the offspring of a mother with long-standing toxoplasmosis infection is considered very low; the exception would be for mothers with a significant degree of immune system disorders.

Q: What is the risk of congenital infection in the offspring of a mother with documented primary infection during pregnancy?
A: Approximately 7–30% of infants born to mothers with active infection during pregnancy are infected themselves.

Tracheitis

 Basics

DESCRIPTION

Tracheitis is inflammation of the trachea, or wind-pipe.
- Acute tracheitis: potentially life-threatening bacterial infection of the trachea, which presents acutely in the otherwise normal child
- Subacute tracheitis: infectious complication of long-term intubation or tracheostomy, primarily in children with an underlying respiratory, neurologic, or other chronic disorder

SIGNS AND SYMPTOMS

- Fever
- Lethargy
- Cough
- Hoarseness
- Noisy breathing
- Anxiety
- Shortness of breath
- Labored breathing
- Bluish discoloration around eyes, lips, and nail beds (cyanosis)

CAUSES

Bacterial or viral infection

SCOPE

- Most common in infancy through early adolescence
- Increased incidence during viral respiratory season

 Diagnosis

QUESTIONS THE DOCTOR MAY ASK

- Immunization history?
- Upper airway infection?
- Fever?
- Cough?
- Exposure to ill people?
- Difficulty breathing?

WHAT THE DOCTOR LOOKS FOR

Signs and symptoms of tracheitis

TESTS AND PROCEDURES

- Tracheal culture
- Blood culture
- Blood tests
- The airway may be examined by laryngoscopy or bronchoscopy.
- X-rays

Treatment

GENERAL MEASURES

- Maintain open airway.
- Provide rescue breathing if needed.
- Drug therapy

ACTIVITY

N/A

DIET

N/A

Medications

COMMONLY PRESCRIBED DRUGS

Antibiotics

Follow-Up

WHAT TO EXPECT

- Patient should improve within 24 to 48 hours unless there are complications.
- Outcome can vary depending on complications.

SIGNS TO WATCH

- Persistent fever
- Sudden worsening of symptoms

PREVENTION

N/A

Common Questions and Answers

Q: Are routing surveillance cultures of patients with artificial airways helpful in prevention or treatment of tracheitis recurrence?
A: No. Children who have been hospitalized and have artificial airways rapidly become colonized with whatever organisms are common within the institution. These organisms will persist for months, are difficult to eradicate, and even if eradicated will be replaced with other, possibly more resistant flora. Routine culture is expensive and will only identify colonization.

Q: Should children with tracheitis be managed in a community hospital or is transfer to a tertiary care center necessary?
A: The most important factor to consider in the initial stages is the availability of someone to ensure an adequate airway (e.g., someone skilled in intubating children) and the presence of someone to closely monitor the patient for decompensation. Once the airway is controlled, the patient should be followed in a setting accustomed to dealing with children requiring mechanical ventilation.

Q: How can you differentiate a child with severe pharyngitis and tracheitis?
A: In many ways, the clinical presentation of tracheitis is similar to that of a severe pharyngitis, bit in tracheitis there will be signs of respiratory compromise (e.g., stridor) and toxic appearance. The two illnesses may look very similar early in the disease course.

Transient Synovitis

 Basics

DESCRIPTION

Transient synovitis is a temporary inflammatory process resulting in joint pain (especially affecting the hip) and occasionally rash precipitated by an exposure to an infectious agent or drug.

SIGNS AND SYMPTOMS

- Pain in joints
- Refusal to bear weight on leg
- Limited range of motion in an extremity
- Rash

CAUSES

Virus, vaccine, drugs (especially antibiotics).

SCOPE

Any age at risk, common in ages 3–10, with males affected 1.5 times more often than females

 Diagnosis

QUESTIONS THE DOCTOR MAY ASK

- Trauma?
- Fever?
- Exercise?
- Sudden onset?
- Recent exposure to a virus, vaccine, drug, or other precipitating agent?

WHAT THE DOCTOR LOOKS FOR

- Joint pain
- Mobility of joint
- Evidence of trauma

TESTS AND PROCEDURES

- Blood tests
- X-rays
- Fluid from joint may be sampled for analysis.

 Treatment

GENERAL MEASURES

N/A

ACTIVITY

N/A

DIET

N/A

Medications

COMMONLY PRESCRIBED DRUGS

- Nonsteroidal anti-inflammatory drugs (NSAIDS)
- Rarely, a short course of oral steroids is necessary.

 ## Follow-Up

WHAT TO EXPECT

- Usually marked improvement in 24 to 48 hours
- Prognosis is excellent, although patients occasionally experience recurrence of symptoms with subsequent viral syndrome or re-exposure to a previously associated drug.

SIGNS TO WATCH

Persistence of symptoms

PREVENTION

N/A

Common Questions and Answers

Q: Is there an association with chronic arthritis?
A: No, there is no known increased risk for chronic arthritis in affected children.

Tuberculosis

 ## Basics

DESCRIPTION

Tuberculosis (TB) is an increasingly common infection in the 1990s. After the tuberculosis organisms take residence in the lung, TB can lead to involvement of multiple other areas of the body, including middle ear, bones, joints, brain, heart, and skin. Organisms can survive many years in the body. The highest risk for active disease is within the first 2 years after exposure.

SIGNS AND SYMPTOMS

- Cough
- Spitting of blood
- Fever and night sweats
- Weight loss
- Decreased activity
- Enlarged lymph glands
- Chest pain

CAUSES

Infection with *Mycobacterium tuberculosis, Mycobacterium bovis,* and *Mycobacterium africanum*

SCOPE

- Congenital infection (acquired from infected mother) occurs rarely.
- Approximately 8% (19 million) Americans have been infected with TB; 45% of these patients are African Americans; 25% are Caucasians over 70 years of age.
- The number of individuals with active contagious disease is approximately 25,000.
- Only 10% of those infected develop the disease, and this is reduced by 60 to 90% if preventive drugs are taken within the first 2 years of infection.
- However, infants, children less than 5 years old, adolescents, and those with a suppressed immune system have higher risks of progression of infection to disease.

 ## Diagnosis

QUESTIONS THE DOCTOR MAY ASK

- Fever?
- Cough?
- Exposure to people with TB or cough?
- Drinking unpasteurized milk?

WHAT THE DOCTOR LOOKS FOR

- The doctor will perform a physical examination to identify the presence of tuberculosis.
- Conditions that can appear similar to TB should be ruled out, including pneumonia, cancer, and fungal infections.

TESTS AND PROCEDURES

- Blood tests
- Special tests for tuberculosis, including sputum culture
- Chest X-ray
- Spinal fluid may be sampled by lumbar puncture (spinal tap).
- A sample of bone marrow may be obtained by biopsy for laboratory analysis.

Treatment

GENERAL MEASURES

- Drug therapy
- Hospitalization may be required for active disease.
- Isolation may be required.

ACTIVITY

N/A

DIET

N/A

 ## Medications

COMMONLY PRESCRIBED DRUGS

- INH
- Rifampin
- Pyrazinamide
- Streptomycin
- Ethambutol

 ## Follow-Up

WHAT TO EXPECT

- Drug therapy may take 2 years or more.
- Cure rate is very high for those who complete course of drug therapy.
- The death rate for untreated TB is 40% over 4 years.
- For outbreaks of drug-resistant tuberculosis, death rates have ranged from 70 to 90%.

PREVENTION

- Tuberculosis screening
- Completion of course of antibiotics (incomplete treatment leads to drug resistance)
- BCG vaccine

SIGNS TO WATCH

N/A

 ## Common Questions and Answers

Q: Why are four drugs necessary for treatment?
A: Even if the organism is sensitive, studies have shown successful short-course anti-TB medication depends on these regimens, especially given the practical difficulties encountered when treating children with any long-term medication.

Q: If the child has completed a course of medication and is re-exposed, what are the risks of infection?
A: One course of preventive therapy is believed to confer immunity to subsequent exposure.

Ulcerative Colitis

 ## Basics

DESCRIPTION

Ulcerative colitis, also called idiopathic proctocolitis, is one of a group of inflammatory bowel diseases of unknown cause characterized by periodic acute episodes of rectal bleeding and various constitutional symptoms.

SIGNS AND SYMPTOMS

- Bloody diarrhea
- Abdominal pain
- Fever
- Weight loss
- Joint pain
- Inflammation of the backbone
- Eye diseases
- Painful nodes on the lower extremities
- Chronic ulcers of the skin
- Mouth ulcers
- Liver and gallbladder disease
- Blood-clotting disorders

CAUSES

The basic cause of ulcerative colitis is unknown. Genetic, infectious, immunologic, and psychological factors have been suggested.

SCOPE

Ulcerative colitis affects 70–150 per 100,000 persons. There are 6–8 new cases per 100,000 population annually in the United States.

MOST OFTEN AFFECTED

- Ulcerative colitis most often affects those between 15 and 35 years of age.
- Average age of onset is 5.9 years.
- Ulcerative colitis tends to run in families; approximately 8–11% of sufferers have a family history of the disease.
- More common in Jews than in other ethnic groups

 ## Diagnosis

QUESTIONS THE DOCTOR MAY ASK

- Rectal bleeding?
- Abdominal pain?
- Weight loss?
- Antibiotic usage?
- Mouth sores?
- Stool pattern?
- Diet?

WHAT THE DOCTOR LOOKS FOR

- Eye examination
- Paleness
- Joint pain
- Abdominal soreness

TESTS AND PROCEDURES

- Blood tests
- Stool analysis
- Abdominal X-ray
- Barium enema
- Upper gastrointestinal (GI) and small bowel series

Treatment

GENERAL MEASURES

- Bowel rest
- Hospitalization may be required.
- Surgery may be needed.
- Drug management

ACTIVITY

N/A

DIET

N/A

 ## Medications

COMMONLY PRESCRIBED DRUGS

- Methylprednisolone
- Prednisone
- Sulfasalazine
- Folic acid
- 5-ASA drugs
- Rowasa enema
- Rowasa suppository
- Hydrocortisone enema
- Hydrocortisone foam
- Cyclosporine
- 6-Mercaptopurine
- Azathioprine

 ## Follow-Up

WHAT TO EXPECT

- The course of the disorder is extremely variable. Approximately 75–85% of patients have a repeat episode of acute illness, and up to 20% may eventually require surgery.
- The risk of death from an initial attack is relatively low—approximately 5% of patients.
- Colon cancer risk is the single most important risk factor affecting long-term prognosis.

SIGNS TO WATCH

- Weight loss
- Abdominal distention
- Mouth sores
- Rectal bleeding

PREVENTION

N/A

 ## Common Questions and Answers

Q: How do you differentiate ulcerative colitis from Chron disease?
A: This is difficult. The combination of blood test, X-rays, and biopsy can usually help make the correct diagnosis.

Q: What is the incidence of cancer in patients with ulcerative colitis?
A: Malignancy rate is 0.5–1% per year a decade after onset. Lifetime, the rate is 15%, three times the normal population.

Urinary Tract Infection

 Basics

DESCRIPTION

A urinary tract infection is an infection of the kidney, bladder, and urethra.

SIGNS AND SYMPTOMS

- Difficult urination
- Hesitancy
- Discomfort in the lower abdomen
- Blood in the urine
- Malodorous urine
- Irritability
- Chills
- Nausea
- Flank pain
- Fever

CAUSES

- Recent urinary tract procedures
- Bacterial infection
- Sexual activity
- Dysfunctional voiding
- Urinary tract abnormalities

SCOPE

Males are most at risk for urinary tract infection during first year of life; females are most at risk until school age and again in adolescence.

 Diagnosis

QUESTIONS THE DOCTOR MAY ASK

- Fever?
- Abdominal pain?
- Painful urination?
- Growth pattern?
- Back pain?
- Malodorus urine?
- Bed wetting?
- Urinary incontinence?

WHAT THE DOCTOR LOOKS FOR

- Irritation of urethra
- Innervation of genital area
- Blood pressure
- Abdominal pain

TESTS AND PROCEDURES

- Urinalysis and culture
- Ultrasound
- Nuclear scan

Treatment

GENERAL MEASURES

Drug therapy

ACTIVITY

N/A

DIET

Encourage fluids.

 Medications

COMMONLY PRESCRIBED DRUGS

Antibiotics

 Follow-Up

WHAT TO EXPECT

Prompt treatment of urinary tract infections reduces the risk of scarring and its effects.

SIGNS TO WATCH

- Recurrence of symptoms
- Hypertension
- Growth

PREVENTION

- Teach correct wiping (front to back) to young children.
- Preventive antibiotics for selected children
- Attention to good voiding habits

 Common Questions and Answers

Q: Do all children require radiologic evaluation after their first UTI?
A: All boys. Any girl with an upper tract infection. All girls less than 3 years.

Q: Can urine obtained from a urine bag be used as a screen to culture babies for UTI?
A: Since fever = UTI = pyelonephritis in young babies and approximatley 10% will have false-negative screening tests (dipstick, U/A) a sterile urine culture should be sent in any baby or girl less 3 years without a documented source of fever.

Vaginal Discharge

 Basics

DESCRIPTION

Vaginal discharge is the secretion produced by the vagina in response to hormonal changes, irritation, or infection. Normal vaginal discharge in newborns and adolescents is termed leukorrhea.

- Physiologic discharge: vaginal and cervical secretions that change with the adolescent's hormonal state. Females may notice an increase in discharge before their menstrual periods.
- Discharge from vaginitis (infection): may be accompanied by odor, itching, and irritation

SIGNS AND SYMPTOMS

- Discharge from vagina
- Itch, irritation

CAUSES

- Pubertal physiologic discharge
- Physiologic discharge
- Bacterial infection
- Chemical vaginitis: soaps, bubble baths, feminine deodorants, and douches
- Foreign bodies: forgotten tampons, condoms, sponges, objects used for masturbation
- Other disease

SCOPE

Physiologic discharge is experienced by most, if not all, pubertal adolescents.

 Diagnosis

QUESTIONS THE DOCTOR MAY ASK

- Do you wipe from back to front?
- Does the discharge get better after your period is finished?
- How long have you noticed the discharge?
- Do you see it in your underwear and/or when you wipe yourself after using the bathroom?

WHAT THE DOCTOR LOOKS FOR

- Relation of discharge to menstrual cycle
- Sexual activity
- Oral contraceptive use
- Medications, including antibiotics and steroids
- History of diabetes mellitus
- Use of douches, feminine deodorants, soaps, or bubble baths
- Use of nylon (noncotton crotch) panties
- Description of discharge: color, consistency, odor
- Presence or absence of vaginal itching
- Method of wiping used by patient after voiding
- Physical examination

TESTS AND PROCEDURES

- Culture for microbiological analysis
- Blood tests

Treatment

GENERAL MEASURES

- Physiologic discharge: education and reassurance
- Foreign body: removal of object
- Chemical vaginitis: discontinuation of irritant

ACTIVITY

N/A

DIET

N/A

 ## Medications

COMMONLY PRESCRIBED DRUGS

Antibiotics

 ## Follow-Up

WHAT TO EXPECT

- Physiologic discharge: continues until menopause
- Vaginitis and cervicitis: improves after specific treatment
- Foreign body: improves after removal of object
- Chemical vaginitis: improves within days after discontinuation of irritant

SIGNS TO WATCH

- Change in color, quality, or amount of discharge
- Vulval swelling
- Abdominal pain
- Vaginal bleeding

PREVENTION

- Wipe from front to back.
- Avoid tight clothing.
- Practice good hygiene.

 ## Common Questions and Answers

Q: How do I know if discharge is normal?
A: Physiologic discharge has no odor, color, or itching.

Q: Should adolescents use douches?
A: No, they are not recommended for adolescents. Douches can strip away the vagina's natural defense mechanisms.

Q: What is the most common finding in a prepubertal girl with a foreign body?
A: Vaginal bleeding alone is the most common finding in vaginal foreign body. The commonly described bloody foul-smelling discharge was seen slightly less often in a recent study.

Ventricular Tachycardia

 ## Basics

DESCRIPTION

Ventricular tachycardia (VT) is a series of heartbeats originating in the ventricle of the heart in excess of 120 beats a minute. It is usually felt as palpitations or light-headedness.

SIGNS AND SYMPTOMS

- May cause no symptoms
- Rapid heart rate
- Palpitations
- Chest pain
- Light-headedness, fainting

CAUSES

- In many cases, the cause is known.
- Heart conditions
- Metabolic disturbances
- Drug ingestion or toxicity
- Central nervous system trauma

SCOPE

- Normal hearts: 0.3–2.2% incidence
- Ventricular tachycardia is very rare in children with normal hearts.

 ## Diagnosis

QUESTIONS THE DOCTOR MAY ASK

- Feeling of rapid heart beat?
- Fainting?
- Difficulty breathing?

WHAT THE DOCTOR LOOKS FOR

- Irregular heart beat
- Heart murmur
- Blood pressure

TESTS AND PROCEDURES

- Electrocardiogram (EKG)
- Cardiac echo
- Holter monitor (usually 48 hours)
- Exercise stress test
- Cardiac catheterization
- Electrophysiology study
- Blood tests

Treatment

GENERAL MEASURES

- Asymptomatic patients with normal hearts only need close follow-up.
- Those with heart disease are usually treated with drugs.
- Surgery may be required.

ACTIVITY

N/A

DIET

N/A

 Medications

COMMONLY PRESCRIBED DRUGS

- Mexiletine
- Beta-blockers
- Quinidine
- Tocainide
- Amiodarone

 Follow-Up

WHAT TO EXPECT

- Outcome is often very good.
- When due to heart disease, outcome depends on the underlying cause.

SIGNS TO WATCH

- Chest pain
- Crying

PREVENTION

N/A

 Common Questions and Answers

Q: Do patients with ventricular tachycardia usually have underlying heart disease?
A: Yes.

Viral Hepatitis

 ## Basics

DESCRIPTION

Viral hepatitis is a group of viral infections involving the liver. Complications range from jaundice to death.

SCOPE

- Hepatitis A virus (HAV): 50% over age 49 have been exposed; HAV is found in 25% of cases of acute hepatitis
- Hepatitis B virus (HBV): approximately 200,000 persons are infected annually. There are more than 500,000 carriers of HBV.
- Hepatitis C virus (HCV): becoming the most common cause of acute and chronic viral hepatitis; 150,000 persons infected annually

SIGNS AND SYMPTOMS

- Fever
- Malaise, fatigue
- Nausea
- Loss of appetite
- Jaundice
- Dark urine
- Abdominal pain
- Headache
- Vomiting

CAUSES

- Viral infection
- Infection may be with multiple different viruses.
- Maximum infectivity 2 weeks before jaundice
- HBV is transmitted sexually, by blood or its products, and during pregnancy.
- HAV is transmitted by the fecal-oral route.

SCOPE

Hepatitis occurs in all ages; rare in infants; susceptibility increases with age.

 ## Diagnosis

QUESTIONS THE DOCTOR MAY ASK

- Exposure to jaundiced patient?
- Immunization of Hepatitis B vaccine?
- Jaundice?
- Dark urine?
- Light-colored stools?
- Travel history?
- Sexual history?

WHAT THE DOCTOR LOOKS FOR

- Jaundice
- Growth failure
- Large liver
- Swelling

TESTS AND PROCEDURES

- Blood tests
- Liver ultrasound
- Computed tomography (CT)
- Liver biopsy

 ## Treatment

GENERAL MEASURES

- Viral hepatitis is usually managed on an out-patient basis.
- Hospitalization may be required.
- Segregation advisable for food handlers or health care workers.
- Acute cases must be reported to public health department.
- Liver transplantation may be necessary.

ACTIVITY

As tolerated

DIET

Adequate calories; balanced nutrition

Medications

COMMONLY PRESCRIBED DRUGS

- Interferon, ribavirin (Virazole)
- Amantadine (Symmetrel)
- Steroids

 Follow-Up

WHAT TO EXPECT

- The outcome varies depending on the virus causing hepatitis.
- Severity of liver disease is a good indicator of outcome.
- May progress to chronic disease

SIGNS TO WATCH

Persistence of symptoms

PREVENTION

N/A

 Common Questions and Answers

Q: If my child has hepatitis A or B, can my other children acquire the disease?
A: HAV is transmitted by the fecal-oral route and can infect family members. HBV is transmitted sexually or through blood products.

Q: My child is on antiseizure medications including Tegretol. Does he need screening liver function tests?
A: Yes.

Von Willebrand Disease

 Basics

DESCRIPTION

Von Willebrand disease is a mild bleeding disorder caused by a defect in certain clotting factors, or the proteins involved in blood clotting.

SIGNS AND SYMPTOMS

- May cause no symptoms
- Bruising
- Nose bleeds
- Excessive menstrual flow
- Other unusual bleeding

CAUSES

Inherited genetic defect

SCOPE

Prevalence in United States is unknown because von Willebrand disease is often very mild. It is believed to affect up to 1% or more of the population.

 Diagnosis

QUESTIONS THE DOCTOR MAY ASK

- Family history of von Willebrand disease or bleeding tendency?
- Bruising?
- Nosebleeds?

WHAT THE DOCTOR LOOKS FOR

- Bleeding patterns
- Physical examination
- Enlarged spleen

TESTS AND PROCEDURES

Blood tests

 Treatment

GENERAL MEASURES

Supportive measures for bleeding

ACTIVITY

Avoid contact sports (football, etc.); otherwise, normal activity for age

DIET

N/A

Medications

COMMONLY PRESCRIBED DRUGS

- DDAVP (desmopressin acetate)
- Blood products

 ## Follow-Up

WHAT TO EXPECT

- Life-long risk of bleeding
- Prognosis is excellent for some forms of the disease; outcome is less favorable for severe forms of the disease.
- With proper education and treatment, patients with the most severe forms of the disease can be expected to do well.

SIGNS TO WATCH

Pattern of bleeding

 ## Common Questions and Answers

Q: How can a child have a bleeding disorder if he/she went through surgery without a problem?
A: In von Willebrand disease, blood clotting factor levels can change as a function of stresses in the body. Many conditions cause the factor level to rise to a normal level. These conditions include infectious illnesses and pregnancy, as well as emotional stress. In surgery, the reason for the surgery itself (e.g., appendicitis, etc.) may cause enough stress to raise the factor levels to normal and prevent bleeding.

Q: Is this bleeding disorder like hemophilia? Will the child get acquired immune deficiency syndrome (AIDS)?
A: von Willebrand disease is not hemophilia. A person is at risk for getting the human immunodeficiency virus (HIV), which causes AIDS, when exposed to infected blood products. Cryoprecipitate and Humate P are both blood products that are used for the treatment of von Willebrand's disease. Fortunately, most patients respond well to a synthetic agent called DDAVP. This medication can be used to prevent bleeding and is not a blood product. In addition, all blood donations are now screened for HIV.

Q: Should the other family members be tested?
A: Yes, even if there is no clear family history. Other affected family members may be unaware that they have the disease because the disease can be so mild.

Warts

 ## Basics

DESCRIPTION

Warts are painless, benign skin tumors characterized by an area of well-defined thickening of the skin. They are caused by a virus passed by direct contact with an infected person or from recently shed virus kept intact in a moist, warm environment. There are many types of warts, with different appearances and growth patterns. Plantar warts are individual or groups or warts that occur on the sole of the foot.

SIGNS AND SYMPTOMS

- Rough-surfaced, raised, skin-colored bumps 1–10 mm in diameter
- Warts may occur individually, in a line, or in a cluster.
- Some warts are a taller, flexible mass of skin resembling cauliflower.
- Some warts are flat and reddish.
- Signs and symptoms of plantar warts include:
  ▸ Individual or grouped warts on the sole of the foot
  ▸ Foot pain
  ▸ Formation of callus
  ▸ Pain in the foot, leg, or back due to distortion of normal posture

CAUSES

Infection with the human papilloma virus (HPV)

SCOPE

- Warts affect 7–10% of population; highest incidence between 10 and 19 years of age; lesions persist for a few months to 5 years.
- 25% of common warts disappear spontaneously in 3 to 6 months; 65% disappear spontaneously by 2 years.
- Plantar warts: spontaneous regression much more common in children than adults; 40% spontaneously regress within 6 months in prepubescent children.

 ## Diagnosis

QUESTIONS THE DOCTOR MAY ASK

- Duration?
- Change in size?
- Medication?

WHAT THE DOCTOR LOOKS FOR

- Presence, distribution, and type of warts
- The doctor will consider other conditions that may appear similar, such as corns, calluses, or scar tissue.

TESTS AND PROCEDURES

- A biopsy of tissue may be obtained for pathologic examination.
- Blood tests

 ## Treatment

GENERAL MEASURES

- If warts cause no symptoms, no treatment is necessary. However, there may be a risk that warts will spread.
- Conservative, nonscarring treatments are preferred.
- Treatment is associated with a 60–70% cure rate.
- Warm soaks followed by peeling the top layer of skin on repeated occasions may speed disappearance.
- Over-the-counter remedies containing salicylic acid may help. Read and follow directions carefully.
- Other measures include use of a heel bar or appropriate padding to relieve pressure points where warts tend to aggregate.

- Occlusion is the easiest and least expensive treatment. The wart is covered with a waterproof tape for a week. The tape is removed and left open for 12 hours, then re-taped if wart is still present. The environment under the tape hinders viral growth.
- Surgical measures include:
  - ▶ Cryotherapy: freezing of warts is often preferred because scar formation is minimized. Usually requires several treatments.
  - ▶ Excision with electrocautery, laser, or curettage
  - ▶ Blunt dissection: a simple surgical procedure that is effective and usually nonscarring; involves separating wart and normal skin with a blunt instrument

ACTIVITY

Plantar warts occasionally cause discomfort, requiring a decrease in activity.

DIET

N/A

 ## Medications

COMMONLY PRESCRIBED DRUGS

- No effective antiviral wart medications currently exist.
- All treatments begin by paring the wart as closely as possible, then soaking the area in warm water to moisten the wart.
- Chemotherapy:
  - ▶ Topical retinoids: tretinoin (retinoic acid, Retin-A)
  - ▶ Salicylic acid (Trans-Ver-Sal, Mediplast, Duofilm, Keralyt)
  - ▶ Formaldehyde
  - ▶ Trichloroacetic
  - ▶ Cantharidin
  - ▶ Podophyllum resin

 ## Follow-Up

WHAT TO EXPECT

- Outcome varies with treatment type.
- Common warts improve slowly over weeks to months. They may resolve spontaneously; remainder resolve with therapy but may have multiple recurrences; children with immune system disorders may have extensive spread of lesions.

SIGNS TO WATCH

N/A

PREVENTION

N/A

 ## Common Questions and Answers

Q: Did my child get these from catching frogs?
A: No, warts are caused by a virus, and he/she probably got them from contact with another child.

Q: Do the warts he/she has in the genital region definitely mean he/she has been sexually abused?
A: No, especially in the first few years of life, warts in the perineal region may represent spread from an infected mother.

Whooping Cough

 ## Basics

DESCRIPTION

Whooping cough, or pertussis, is a highly contagious respiratory infection. It causes a characteristic cough that ends in a high-pitched whoop or crow.

SIGNS AND SYMPTOMS

- Spasms of cough
- "Whoop" cough
- Inhale "gasp" or vomiting after cough
- Mild fever
- Runny nose
- Loss of appetite
- Episodes of apnea

CAUSES

Infection with *Bordetella pertussis* bacteria

SCOPE

- Whooping cough is a disease of young children; infants and children with a compromised immune system are at greatest risk.
- Approximately one-third of cases reported to the Centers for Disease Control are in infants less than 6 months old.
- Disease in adolescents and adults is not usually recognized as whooping cough and may last for weeks. These patients are the major source of pertussis infection in children.

 ## Diagnosis

QUESTIONS THE DOCTOR MAY ASK

- Immunization history?
- Exposure?
- Vomiting at end of cough?
- Cyanosis?
- Characteristic "whoop" cough?

WHAT THE DOCTOR LOOKS FOR

- Typical stages of illness development
- Physical examination

TESTS AND PROCEDURES

- Blood tests
- Chest X-ray
- Culture for microbiological analysis

 ## Treatment

GENERAL MEASURES

- Patients with more severe disease or other complications require hospitalization for supportive care.
- Antibiotics

ACTIVITY

N/A

DIET

N/A

Medications

COMMONLY PRESCRIBED DRUGS

- Erythromycin, trimethoprim-sulfamethoxazole
- Corticosteroids and beta-agonist aerosols

Follow-Up

WHAT TO EXPECT

- The prognosis is directly related to patient age; the highest death rate is in infants less than 6 months of age.
- Infants have a 0.5–1% risk of death whereas, in the older child, prognosis is good.
- The spasms of cough can last up to 4 weeks and the convalescence stage up to several months and can be quite problematic for patient and family.
- The complications of whooping cough are more likely to occur in the younger infant, and infants therefore tend to have a more serious, protracted course.

SIGNS TO WATCH

N/A

PREVENTION

- Pertussis vaccine
- Respiratory isolation for 5 days after starting antibiotic therapy or until at least 3 weeks after the onset of the spasm cough stage, if antibiotics were not given, is recommended.
- Exposed individuals (all household contacts, other close contacts, other children in child care) should receive preventive antibiotics to limit transmission.

Common Questions and Answers

Q: Are ther any risks associated with the pertussis vaccine?
A: There are local and febrile reactions that are common to the DTP vaccine; anaphylaxis is estimated to occur in 2 cases/100,000 injections; risk of seizures occurring within 48 hours of administration is 1:1750 doses and is believed to be due to a febrile seizure; inconsolable crying for 3 or more hours is observed in 1:100 doses given; a hypertonic-hyporesponsive episode occurs in 1:1750 doses. Because of the temporal relation between administration of pertussis vaccine and severe adverse events such as death, encephalopathy, developmental delay with learning and behavioral problems or onset of seizures, much publicity has been given to this vaccine, yet causation has not been established.

Q: What are the contraindications to pertussis vaccination?
A: Contraindications to avoid initial or subsequent doses of pertussis vaccine include the following: immediate anaphylactic reaction, encephalopath within 7 days of a prior injection or a seizure within 3 days or persistent crying, a shock-like state or fever greater than 104.9°F within 48 hours of a prior injection. A progressive neurologic disorder or history of seizure disorder are contraindications also.

Yersinia Enterocolitica

 Basics

DESCRIPTION

Yersinia enterocolitica is a bacterium that produces a diarrheal disease.

SIGNS AND SYMPTOMS

- Diarrhea that may contain blood or mucus
- Fever
- Abdominal pain
- Joint pain

CAUSES

Bacterial infection

SCOPE

- Most infected individuals are young children.
- *Y. enterocolitica* has been isolated from contaminated water, soil, wild and domestic animals, and unpasteurized milk products.
- The incubation period is approximately 1–11 days with symptoms persisting for 5 to 14 days.
- Symptoms lasting up to several months have been reported.

 Diagnosis

QUESTIONS THE DOCTOR MAY ASK

- Exposure to unpasteurized milk?
- Abdominal pain?
- Description of diarrhea?
- Fever?

WHAT THE DOCTOR LOOKS FOR

- Examination is usually normal.
- Tenderness in abdomen

TESTS AND PROCEDURES

- Culture for microbiological analysis
- Blood tests
- Stool analysis

 Treatment

GENERAL MEASURES

Antibiotics

ACTIVITY

N/A

DIET

N/A

Medications

COMMONLY PRESCRIBED DRUGS

Antibiotics

Follow-Up

WHAT TO EXPECT

- Symptoms usually abate within 2 weeks, although shedding of the organism in the stool can last at least 6 weeks after diagnosis.
- The expected course is dependent on the specific organ system involved.
- The prognosis is usually quite good.
- Systemic disease causes more severe illness and greater risk of death.

SIGNS TO WATCH

N/A

PREVENTION

- Infection control: precautions are indicated for patients with enterocolitis until symptoms resolve.
- General measures: Avoid ingesting contaminated foods and beverages, uncooked meats (especially pork) and unpasteurized milk; avoid preparation of meats near or during preparation of infant bottles for feeding.

Common Questions and Answers

Q: How long is a child considered infectious with *Y. enterocolitica?*
A: Although the typical course of enterocolitis is approximately 14 days, shedding of the organism in the stool can last at least 6 weeks.

SECTION II:
Definitions

Definitions

Anemia of chronic disease—Anemia accompanying inflammation, infection or other chronic disease; therapy is directed at underlying disease; treatment may include transfusion or drug.

Aplastic anemia—Bone marrow disorder; failure of bone marrow to make red cells, most cases of unknown cause; produces weakness, fatigue, bleeding disorders; treated with bone marrow transplantation or drugs; can be fatal if untreated, but with treatment most people recover within 70 to 100 days.

Ascites—Accumulation of fluid in the abdomen resulting from low serum protein or increased venous pressure; may be related to heart or liver disease; treatment is directed at underlying disease.

Biliary atresia—A progressive disease of the bile ducts that produces jaundice and liver failure in infants; few cases may be corrected by surgery or transplantation; can result in long-term complications.

Botulism—Nerve damage caused by a toxin produced by the bacterium *Clostridium botulinum*; results in breathing failure, constipation, muscle weakness, paralysis; potentially life-threatening condition requiring hospitalization.

Cataract—Cloudiness of the eye lens, resulting in impaired vision; treated with surgical extraction; life-long treatment and follow-up required.

Cirrhosis—Liver disease caused by viral infection or other insults; may produce metabolic problems or bleeding disorders; treatment includes drugs and surgery; outcome depends on cause.

Condyloma accumulata—Venereal or genital warts; may be surgically removed, but tend to recur.

Costochondritis—Chest pain caused by inflammation of rib cartilage; pressing on ribs makes pain worse; treated with nonsteroidal analgesics and rest; antibiotics may be prescribed if infection present; prognosis is usually excellent.

Cutaneous larva migrans—Infection of skin by nematode usually transmitted from dogs and cats; produces intensely itchy, raised lines in skin; treated with freezing of skin.

Diabetic ketoacidosis—Severe metabolic disorder affecting those with diabetes; associated with high blood sugar; produces weight loss, excessive thirst and urination, nausea, vomiting, lethargy, fruity odor to breath; usually requires hospitalization; treated with insulin and other medications; can cause serious complications but in most cases recovery is good.

Diskitis—Inflammation of a disk of the spinal column; causes discomfort, rigid posture, refusal to walk, fever, back or abdominal pain; treated with nonsteroidal anti-inflammatory drugs (NSAIDs); prognosis is usually excellent.

Erythema multiforme—A red skin rash of many forms; careful observation will find dark, target-shaped or ring-like lesions; often preceded by fever and malaise; mild forms are self-limiting; severe forms may require drugs and more intensive treatment.

Ewing sarcoma—Bone cancer causing pain, swelling, fever, pack pain and paralysis of the lower extremities; treated with surgery, radiation, and chemotherapy; 50–70% of patients can be cured.

Fungal skin infections—May affect skin, hair, or nails; includes ringworm, cradle cap, and candidiasis; treated with topical or oral antifungal medication; outcome is generally good, but infection often recurs.

Growth hormone deficiency—Hormone disorder leading to short stature, delay in puberty, and other systemic effects; treated with replacement of hormone.

Hereditary spherocytosis—Inherited anemia with round cells—spherocytes.

Hirschsprung disease—Lower intestinal obstruction caused by absence of nerve cells in intestinal wall producing a narrow segment in uterus; main symptom is constipation with overflow diarrhea; treated with surgery.

Hodgkin lymphoma—Enlargement of the lymph glands; most commonly painless; may cause fatigue, loss of appetite, weight loss; treated with radiation and chemotherapy.

Definitions

Intussusception—"Telescoping" of one portion of intestine into another; produces colic-like pain, vomiting, blood and mucus in stool; usually reduced by barium enema but surgery may be required.

Meckel diverticulum—An abnormal segment of stomach cells producing acid; found in small bowel; may cause intermittent painless rectal bleeding, abdominal pain, and intestinal obstruction; treated with surgery.

Megaloblastic anemia—Anemia characterized by large red cells; usually caused by folic acid or vitamin B_{12} deficiency; may cause pallor, fatigue, poor appetite, irritability, gastrointestinal disturbances, and neurological symptoms; treated with folic acid or vitamin B_{12}.

Metabolic disease in newborns—Inborn metabolic disorders often are apparent within 10 days of birth; may cause a characteristic odor in urine or other body fluids, abnormal growth, abnormal muscle tone, seizures or changes in consciousness, and other symptoms; treatment and outcome depend on cause.

Munchausen syndrome by proxy—The persistent fabrication of child's symptoms given by parent, causing that person to be regarded as ill; unexplained medical illnesses (usually infections, sudden respiratory failure), apparently ineffective treatment are clues; psychotherapy for parent is warranted.

Muscular dystrophy—Hereditary disorder causing progressive weakness and degeneration of muscle; treatment is mainly supportive; medications not effective; genetic counseling and support groups are recommended.

Myasthenia gravis—Variable and intermittent weakness and fatigue of muscle that is worse with activity and better with rest; supportive care and medications; outcome is variable; some forms have a high death rate.

Nephrotic syndrome—Kidney disorder caused by loss of protein in urine; produces weight gain and facial swelling, abdominal pain and swelling; treated with corticosteroids; resolves over 2 to 4 weeks but recurs many times in most cases; outcome is good in 90% of patients.

Neuroblastoma—A cancer of nerve cells of unknown cause; symptoms depend on body area affected; may affect breathing or digestion; treated with surgery, radiation, chemotherapy, bone marrow transplantation; children with low-risk disease have 85–90% cure rate, while older children with more advanced disease have a lower cure rate.

Non-Hodgkin lymphoma—Cancer of the lymphatic system that is the third most common cancer of childhood; may cause abdominal mass, enlarged lymph nodes, or other symptoms depending on body area affected; treated with radiation, surgery, and chemotherapy; early cancer often has a favorable prognosis.

Osteosarcoma—Cancer affecting bone and other tissues that causes pain and swelling of affected area; treated with surgery and chemotherapy; many children with osteosarcoma of extremity without lung involvement can be cured.

Pancreatitis—Inflammation of the pancreas that typically causes abdominal pain that is made worse by eating; also causes nausea and vomiting; treatment requires hospitalization; rarely leads to chronic pancreatitis.

Perirectal abscess—A localized infection near the rectal area; causes throbbing pain, redness, swelling, tenderness; treated by surgical draining, antibiotics, sitz bath; recovery is usually good.

Persistent pulmonary hypertension of the newborn—Elevated blood pressure in the pulmonary (lung) blood circulation; most common during the first hours after birth; may lead to lung, heart, or central nervous system disorders; requires hospitalization; prognosis is usually good.

Pneumocystis carinii pneumonia—Fungal pneumonia that is the most common opportunistic infection among those with an impaired immune system; respiratory distress, cough, fever, poor feeding, diarrhea; treated with medication; 10–40% death rate among treated patients.

Portal hypertension—Elevated pressure in liver and veins connecting liver and spleen;

Definitions

may cause bleeding in the esophagus, enlarged spleen, and bleeeding; hospitalization may be required; treated with surgery and medication; outcome depends on cause.

Posterior urethral valves—Found in males and located in tube from bladder through penis; folds of tissue that act as valves, leading to obstruction of the urinary system; produces renal failure, labored breathing, and growth failure; the most common form of lower urinary tract obstruction; treated with surgery; outcome is widely variable.

Primary adrenal insufficiency—A congenital deficiency of the production of cortisol and other hormones of adrenal gland, causing weakness and fatigue, loss of appetite, weight loss, headache, nausea, vomiting, abdominal pain, muscle and joint aches, mood swings, salt cravings, and other symptoms; treated with medication; outcome is often good.

Prune belly syndrome—A condition marked by absence or weakness of abdominal muscles, undescended testicles, and dilated ureter (tube connecting kidney to bladder); may be other birth defects; supportive therapy; surgery may be recommended; those that survive the neonatal period have a good prognosis.

Pulmonary embolism—Blockage of a blood vessel in the lung by a blood clot; causes chest pain, shortness of breath, cough, spitting of blood, and other symptoms; requires hospitalization; treated with anticoagulants.

Renal failure, acute—A rapidly progressive cessation of normal kidney function caused by poisons, dehydration, low blood pressure, infections, and other problems; may be associated with fever, rash, bloody diarrhea, vomiting, pallor, absent or scanty volume of urine, hypotension; hospitalization required; treated with medication.

Renal failure, chronic—A reduction of kidney function that causes malaise, poor appetite, vomiting, bone pain, headache, and an excessive volume of urine; treated with medication; dialysis or transplantation may be required.

Retropharyngeal abscess—A rare but potentially dangerous localized infection of the deep tissues in the back of the throat; causes fever, noisy breathing, drooling, tender neck, limited range of motion of the neck; may be medical emergency; hospitalization required; treated with antibiotics and surgery in some cases.

Rhabdomyosarcoma—Cancer involving muscle tissue; causes painless, firm swelling or lump; other symptoms depend on site of lesion; treatment includes surgery and chemotherapy.

Staphylococcal scalded skin syndrome—A bacterial infection of the skin that appears similar to burn injuries; causes fever and skin blisters; treated with antibiotics; prognosis is often good, but outcome is guarded in infants and those with other emdical problems.

Stevens-Johnson syndrome—An allergic reaction marked by a blistered rash, fever, and constitutional symptoms; hospitalization may be required; surgery may be needed; recovery may take weeks; prognosis is often good.

Supraventricular tachycardia—Excessively fast heart rhythm that causes palpitations, dizziness, chect pain, fainting, breathing difficulties, irritability, decreased feedings, decreased urine output; treated with medication; likely to be recur in future.

Tetralology of Fallot—A complex group of heart defects (connection between two lower chambers of heart, abnormal placement of aorta, narrowing of pulmonary valve) that is often detected soon after birth; cyanosis and heart failure corrected by surgery and medication; outcome is often very good.

Tick fever—An infectious disease marked by repalsing fever, chills, headache, muscle aches, rash and other symptoms; treated with removal of tick, antibiotics, and supportive care; prognosis is usually good.

Toxic shock syndrome—An acute bacterial infection marked by muscle pain, diarrhea, sore throat, peeling skin, and other symptoms; may lead to shock or other severe complications; hospitalization required; treated with antibiotics.

Urethral prolapse—The outpouching of the urinary tract through the external opening at the genitalia; treated with antibiotics, sitz bath, topical estrogen; often spontaneously resolves.

Uteropelvic junction obstruction—A blockage of the urinary system near the kidney; may cause fever, flank or back pain, urinary tract infection, blood in urine; corrected with surgery.

Wilms tumor—Cancer of the kidney causing anemia, fever, high blood pressure, and other symptoms; treated with surgery, radiation, and chemotherapy; cure rate ranges from 80% to more than 90%.

Index

Index

Index